Fundamental Techniques of Pla

The Author

Ian A. McGregor

Honorary Clinical Lecturer in Plastic Surgery, University of Glasgow. Consultant Plastic Surgeon, Regional Plastic Surgery Unit, Canniesburn Hospital, Glasgow. Consultant Plastic Surgeon, Royal Infirmary and Western Infirmary, Glasgow.

Foreword by

Sir Charles Illingworth

Emeritus Regius Professor of Surgery, University of Glasgow.

Fundamental Techniques of Plastic Surgery

AND THEIR SURGICAL APPLICATIONS

Ian A. McGregor
M.B., Ch.M., F.R.C.S. (Eng.), F.R.C.S. (Glasg.), Hon. F.R.A.C.S.

Foreword by
Sir Charles Illingworth
C.B.E., M.D., Ch.M., F.R.C.S. (Glasg.), F.R.C.S. (Edin.), Hon. F.A.C.S.,
Hon. F.R.C.S. (Eng.)

SEVENTH EDITION

CHURCHILL LIVINGSTONE
EDINBURGH LONDON AND NEW YORK 1980

CHURCHILL LIVINGSTONE
Medical Division of the Longman Group Limited

Distributed in the United States of America by Churchill
Livingstone Inc., 19 West 44th Street, New York, N.Y.
10036, and by associated companies, branches and rep-
resentatives throughout the world.

First edition 1960
Second edition 1962
Third edition 1965
Fourth edition 1968
Fifth edition 1972
Sixth edition 1975
Seventh edition 1980
Translated into Spanish

ISBN 0 443 01828 6

British Library Cataloguing in Publication Data
McGregor, Ian Alexander
    Fundamental techniques of plastic surgery
    and their surgical applications.–7th ed.
    1. Surgery, Plastic
    I. Title
    617'.95   RD118   79–42717

Printed in Great Britain at The Pitman Press, Bath

Foreword

Like other surgical specialties, Plastic Surgery originated through the efforts of a small group of enthusiasts who, by utilising a particular refinement of technique, soon raised the standards of surgical craftsmanship within a narrow field to a high pitch of efficiency.

Then came the war, and the techniques primarily evolved for hiding facial blemishes and correcting visible deformities were applied with immense success to the treatment of wounds in general. Since then, as a natural sequel, plastic surgeons have widened still further their range of interests, notably in casualty work, in hand injuries and in burns. In doing so, they have implicitly ceased to regard themselves as a class apart, exclusive authorities in a chosen field, but rather as expert advisers and helpful collaborators in a wide range of surgery.

Mr McGregor is emphatically of this latter class, trained in the Glasgow School of Plastic Surgery, broadened in experience by the responsibility of a busy casualty department, and with a particular interest in the surgery of the hand. His book reflects these interests and this experience, being designed not for specialists but for all those who are concerned with the healing of wounds. Its approach is essentially practical, dealing as it does with the choice of incisions, with stitchcraft, avoidance of ugly scars, methods of skin grafting, and similar matters, and with their application to casualty surgery, orthopaedics and general surgery. It will assuredly receive a warm welcome.

Glasgow, 1960.   C. F. W. Illingworth

Preface to the Seventh Edition

The most striking change in this edition is the inclusion of a chapter on muscle and myocutaneous flaps. Muscle flaps did receive mention in the last edition but extension of the technique to include the overlying skin in the transfer, in the form of a myocutaneous flap, has greatly increased its scope and usage, to the extent that it now merits more detailed consideration. Inclusion of these techniques has also made it necessary to be more specific in nomenclature than in the past and refer to flaps which consist of skin and superficial fascia as skin flaps.

Attitudes to skin flaps themselves have also changed, with a much greater concern to exploit their axial vascular elements. This has resulted in a reduction in the popularity of random pattern flaps generally. These changes in emphasis have created problems of exposition. It was previously possible to discuss direct flaps and tube pedicles as the norm, taking the view that axial pattern flaps, which of course share many techniques established in random flap usage such as the tubing of bridge segments and use of the wrist carrier, were merely departures from the norm. But axial pattern flaps are now the norm and the tube pedicle has almost been relegated to 'dinosaur' status. It has been necessary as a result to recast the entire chapter.

The situation in muscle flaps is now relatively stable with those which combine the maximum therapeutic value with the minimum of disability from loss of use of the donor muscle firmly established.

New myocutaneous flaps on the other hand are still appearing in the journals. Selection has been needed to pick the likely winners, viewing the field as a realist rather than as an enthusiast.

These obvious changes apart, the entire book has been subjected to scrutiny with changes of detail and emphasis in several chapters. A considerable number of new illustrations have been required. The drawings are recognisably the work of Mr Robin Callander; the photographs were prepared by Mr Alan McIlroy and the staff of the photography unit at Canniesburn Hospital. The illustrations of the soleus muscle transfer were provided by Mr Martyn H. C. Webster. My secretary, Mrs A. M. Allanach, converted a mixture of new manuscript and minor text changes into a state suitable for presentation to the publishers. To all of these I am most grateful.

Glasgow, 1980   Ian A. McGregor

Preface to the First Edition

Plastic surgical methods are being used increasingly often by surgeons who have received no formal training in plastic surgery and who are looking for guidance on the basic techniques. Advanced textbooks of plastic surgery are apt to pass over those elementary but nonetheless fundamental methods while the sections on plastic surgery in textbooks of surgery describe its scope and results without giving enough detail of actual technique to be of practical use. This book I hope may help to fill the gap.

The first part describes the basic techniques of plastic surgery in detail and the second considers their application to the situations which surgeons in other specialties are likely to encounter. A difficulty in the second part has been that of deciding what material to include and what to leave out. The deciding factor generally has been to include such topics and techniques as it was felt a surgeon in the particular field might reasonably wish to deal with himself without necessarily referring the patient to a plastic surgeon.

The book makes no attempt to describe all possible methods of repair and reconstruction. To include a multiplicity of methods in a book of this nature would merely confuse and I have preferred instead to describe those methods which I have found work best in practice.

In discussing the basic techniques I have tried to stress the difficulties of each and to describe the complications, how they can be avoided and how to cope with them when they do occur. I have endeavoured too, to bring out the principles of the various methods in the hope that an understanding of these principles may weld the technical details into a coherent, rational pattern and prevent them from being a mere jumble of empirical instructions.

A difficult decision has been whether or not to use the eponyms in which plastic surgery abounds. Eponyms are an essential part of everyday surgical shorthand and they recall men who have stood as signposts along the way of an advancing specialty. But often they lack precise meaning and they are liable to cause confusion, firstly because they sometimes have different meanings in different countries, secondly because they are frequently used loosely so that in some instances a name has even come to be applied to a procedure different from that described by its owner. The Thiersch graft is an example of this latter category, being nowadays applied to a graft of quite different thickness from that originally described by Thiersch. For these reasons I have regretfully avoided eponyms altogether.

References have purposely not been introduced into the text. Instead I have listed a few papers and monographs at the end of each chapter under suitable subject headings to provide a starting point for anyone wishing to pursue a particular subject further.

I must acknowledge my debt to many who have helped me in preparing this book. To Professor C. F. W. Illingworth who encouraged me at the outset in its writing and Mr J. S. Tough who was responsible for my training in Plastic Surgery and gave me free access to the photographic records of the Unit I am deeply grateful. I am greatly in debt of Mr Douglas R. K. Reid for his constructive criticism of the text and for the pains he has taken to make it as lucid as possible without sacrificing brevity in the process. To Professor Roland Barnes and Dr J. C. J. Ives who read and criticised parts of the text I express my thanks.

The illustrations are all-important in a book largely concerned with surgical techniques. Mr Robin Callander made all the drawings and I find it difficult to convey fully the care and trouble he has taken to portray visually what I wished to express. Any usefulness which the book may have is due in no small way to his illustrations. The photographs are the work of Mr T. Meikle and Mr R. Macgregor of the Plastic Surgery Units at Ballochmyle Hospital and Glasgow Royal Infirmary; Mr R. McLean, Department of Medical Illustration, Western Infirmary; Mr P. Kelly, Photographic Department and Mr E. Towler, Department of Surgery, Glasgow Royal Infirmary. For the care and trouble which each has taken I am most grateful. I am also indebted to Messrs Chas. F. Thackray for permission to use illustrations of their instruments.

The typing and retyping of the manuscript was carried out with patience and good humour by Mrs A. M. Drummond.

I should like lastly to record my thanks to Mr Charles Macmillan and Mr James Parker of Messrs E. And S. Livingstone for the advice and help which they have given me throughout.

Glasgow, 1960.   Ian A. McGregor

Contents

PART ONE

Basic techniques

1

Wound care

Given accurate skin approximation and freedom from infection epidermal healing occurs extremely rapidly but the healing processes which go on in the dermis are much more prolonged and as far as the ultimate appearance of the resulting scar is concerned far more important. The transition from fibrin, formed between the two surfaces of the wound as the first stage of healing, to the quiescent relatively avascular scar takes place slowly over a period of months.

Early on, the scar tends to be red and the immediate surroundings are indurated, almost wooden, in consistency. Gradually the induration and redness diminish and disappear leaving a soft scar, paler than the surrounding skin. The degree of redness and induration is extremely variable as is the time taken for the reaction to subside; three months to almost a year are the extremes. The appearance of a scar can be expected to improve up to a year and at least the greater part of the reaction should be allowed to subside before secondary revision is considered.

This gradually diminishing induration constitutes normal progress to quiescence. Such a sequence is by no means invariable and instead the fibrous tissue of the dermis may become grossly hypertrophic giving rise clinically to a raised, red, *hypertrophic* scar or when the reaction is more florid to a *keloid* scar, but these conditions are sufficiently important to merit separate consideration.

During the healing phase the tensile strength of the wound gradually increases. The sutures take what little strain there is until they are removed and if a scar is going to stretch it does so gradually over the next few weeks. Support of the wound for as long as is feasible appears to have little effect. Naturally a scar is more likely to stretch badly when skin has been lost and there is obvious wound tension, but often stretching occurs when there is no apparent tension other than that deriving from the normal elasticity of the skin.

Nevertheless in many parts of the body the direction of the scar appears to influence the amount of stretching which takes place and the directions which result in minimal stretching can be systematised into **lines of election for scars**.

In the face and neck the lines of election are at right angles to the direction of the resultant pull of the muscles of facial expression and with the loss of elasticity that goes with ageing they become set into a pattern of wrinkles (Fig. 1.1). In the vicinity of the flexures the lines of election are parallel to the skin creases which are clearly present in the region of the flexure.

In the skin surfaces between the flexures the evidence for a specific line of election is less clear cut and in any case the placing of an incision there is determined more often by considerations other than the eventual cosmetic result of the scar.

In general then an incision should be placed in a line of election where at all possible.

At the outset it must be said that there is great and uncontrollable individual variation in healing characteristics. Examples of factors beyond the surgeon's control are the age of the patient, the site and often the direction of the wound or incision. Scars in children generally remain harder and redder for longer than in the adult and the end result is poorer, this quite apart from the tendency of scars in childhood to develop hypertrophic change or even keloid. One of the compensations of age is the fact that the more wrinkled the skin the more rapidly a scar settles and the better is its final appearance.

Scars also behave very differently in different parts of the body. Outside the face and neck, scars are apt to stay conspicuous despite careful surgical technique and late stretching even of the most meticulously handled incision is frequent. In the face too, different sites and different skins vary greatly in behaviour. Coarse, oily skin tends to produce more than the usual reaction to suture materials and suture marks are the more common as a result. This problem arises most strikingly in the nose where the skin can be very thick with active sebaceous glands, most marked towards the tip. Hairless skin, on the contrary, such as the red margin of the lips and the palms and soles, usually gives less conspicuous scars.

Probably the best example of the influence of direction on scar behaviour is seen in the neck where the horizontal thyroidectomy scar does uniformly well while the vertical scar in the same area does uniformly badly. Equally the best example of the influence of site is the upper sternal area where scars almost invariably become keloid.

Despite these unavoidable factors which set a limit to what can be achieved by pure surgical technique it is nonetheless true that to produce the best result in a given set of circumstances a meticulous technique is essential and it must be emphasised that failure in a single aspect is enough to give a poor result.

The factors concerned in wound care are:

1. Placing the scar
2. Preparing the wound
3. Stitchcraft
4. Postoperative care

An added factor which influences surgical method throughout is the all important need to prevent *haematoma* in wounds.

PLACING THE SCAR

When the onus of placing the scar lies with the surgeon the principles to be followed in selecting site and direction are:

Use of natural lines

The scar should be placed in the line of a wrinkle or at least parallel to it (Fig. 1.1) so that in course of time it will settle in to look like another wrinkle. Even if wrinkling is not actually present, the eventual site of the wrinkles which will develop in the future and, more important, their direction can often be found by getting the patient to simulate the appropriate facial expression, e.g. smiling, frowning, closing the eyelids tightly, etc. This brings the more obvious wrinkle lines into being.

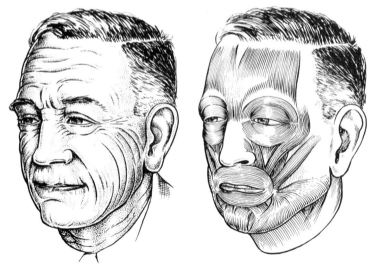

Fig. 1.1 The lines of election for scars in the face and neck shown by the pattern of wrinkling and their relation to the direction of the underlying muscles.

The most generally useful wrinkles develop in relation to the eyes and the mouth—the naso-labial fold, the glabellar wrinkle pattern, the lateral canthal 'crow's foot', the forehead wrinkles. As can be seen (Fig. 1.1) these sites overlie the main concentrations of facial muscle. Where there is less facial muscle, as over the masseter, the wrinkle pattern is less clear cut and in the ear and nasal tip where there is none it is completely lacking.

In the adult the presence of a submandibular 'jowl' associated with slackness of the adjoining skin often creates a superadded wrinkle pattern and this can also be made use of on occasion. Such wrinkling, arising from the effect of gravity on a background of skin slackness, occurs also to a varying degree elsewhere on the face. Indeed in many ageing faces the criss-cross of fine wrinkling is a mixture of gravity wrinkling and expression lines.

In the child with completely smooth skin it can be extremely difficult, especially away from the eyes and mouth, to select the best line for a scar.

In the ear the contour lines of the pinna are useful and they camouflage scars very effectively but for the nasal tip there are really no useful rules to help in selecting the best line.

Where there is a natural junction to distract the eye from a scar this may be used. Examples of these are the junction lines between nose and face especially around the base of the ala, the nostril rim, the margin between the red border of the lip and the skin, the junction line between the ear and the masseteric region, and in the lower eyelid just below the line of the eyelashes. All of these and others are used routinely to distract the eye and render the scar less conspicuous.

Placing the scar where it will not be visible
The obvious examples are inside the hair line or in the eyebrow, and these are the only sites where an incision which is not perpendicular to the skin surface is permissible. Instead the incision should be made parallel to the hair follicles to avoid the hairless scar which sectioning hair follicles would cause. The eyebrow incision is especially useful in approaching a dermoid cyst of the lateral canthal region and the invisible scar more than compensates for the added technical difficulty of such an indirect approach. One practical point to note is the possibility of subsequent baldness revealing a scar previously hidden in the scalp. Account should always be taken of the patient's sex and any hereditary factors in assessing the desirability of using an incision inside the hair line and the precise details of siting.

Use of the Z-plasty

The Z-plasty plays an extremely important part as an adjunct to other methods designed to minimise scars. It is carried out during the excision of a scar by transposing the flaps resulting from two additional side cuts, each made at an angle which may vary but which tends to be in the vicinity of 60°. The effect of this is to alter the line of at least part of the scar and it can be designed so that the alteration brings the line into a wrinkle or line of election.

It is a precise procedure which must be fully understood if it is to be used properly; it is also used in contexts other than those relating to facial scars. In its several contexts it still retains a basic unity of theory and practice and because of this it is convenient to discuss it as a topic on its own in chapter 2.

At this stage it can nevertheless be stated that it should not be used in the primary treatment of wounds resulting from trauma unless the wound approximates in character to a surgical incision and the circumstances are otherwise ideal. Even then it is a procedure for the experienced surgeon. It is better reserved for use in any subsequent scar revision.

PREPARATION OF THE WOUND

When a wound is already present as a result for example of trauma it is important to consider how and to what extent it transgresses the principles of placing a scar and whether it can be modified to fit those principles. It often proves impossible or undesirable to make it conform as a primary manoeuvre because of potential infection, poor blood supply of wound margins, skin damage, etc. and the aim should be to prepare it for the time when, at a later date, it can be modified to conform.

Wounds can be regarded as **traumatised** when the wound edges have been appreciably damaged or **non-traumatised** when the wound edges contain minimal damaged tissue as in surgically created wounds.

It is the presence or absence of damaged tissue which determines whether or not a wound should be excised. Under all circumstances it is axiomatic that all dirt and other foreign material must be removed, by excision if necessary. In the face where the cosmetic result is of paramount importance the problem of excisional policy is more difficult than elsewhere and there are two approaches to the problem:

If damage is minimal the wound may be excised so converting it to an atraumatic type in an attempt to get a final result primarily. This approach is satisfactory only under optimal conditions. If the result is not acceptable, however, the situation can always be retrieved by secondary scar excision provided too much skin has not been excised in the first instance.

In more extensive wounds (Fig. 1.2) the approach is more conservative and only dirt and obviously non-viable tissues are removed. In these circumstances one accepts the need for further surgery in the knowledge that a good scar cannot be expected from the healing of such a wound. This policy permits the salvage of tissue which might otherwise be excised, tissue which may be valuable later.

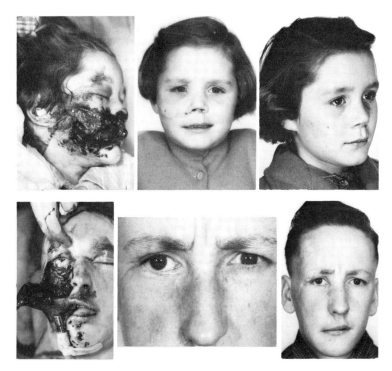

Fig. 1.2 The conservative treatment of severe soft tissue injuries of face involving eyelids, nose, and mouth where there is no skin loss, showing the results of accurate tissue replacement with careful matching.

A conservative policy is obligatory in the care of severe facial soft tissue trauma where it is seldom possible to achieve final reconstruction at the primary operation and where the over-riding object must be to replace structures in their normal position and suture them there. The secret in suturing an irregular wound is to look first for landmarks on either side to match. With two points which definitely fit sutured together fresh parts of the jigsaw fall into place until enough key points have been matched to allow the intervening sutures to be placed readily. Time spent fitting a jigsaw of tissue accurately at the time of original suture is never wasted. The chance comes only once and if it is missed the results can be disastrous. Although it may be quite obvious that Z-plasties will be required later, these should seldom be used at the primary operation.

An added difficulty arises when there has been actual loss of tissue and the governing principle then is to replace surviving tissues in their correct anatomical position so that the defect can be properly displayed and assessed in terms of tissues lost.

While the experienced plastic surgeon may legitimately carry out a primary definitive repair in such circumstances the less experienced surgeon should be more modest and if the defect cannot be closed by direct suture he should apply a split-skin graft in most instances. A full-thickness defect opening into the mouth which cannot be closed without undue distortion calls for suture of skin to mucosa.

These temporary measures have at least the merit of allowing rapid healing with minimal scarring and leave conditions suitable for a definitive repair subsequently.

The common errors in treating wounds at this stage are:

1. Failure to remove all dirt from the wound leaving an area of tattooed scarring (Fig. 1.3) which is usually difficult and often impossible to eradicate later.

2. The production of a scar with gross suture marks (Fig. 1.4). Such a wound would often do better to heal by granulation for the resulting scar however ugly can always be excised. The presence of suture marks, however, makes excision infinitely more difficult.

3. Failure to suture the various wound edges in the precise position which they occupied relative to one another before the injury (Fig. 1.5). The resulting irregularities are especially obvious when the lip margin, eyelid, eyebrow or nostril have been imperfectly matched.

It is often important to know when a piece of traumatised tissue can safely be conserved or whether it must be excised. In deciding this the important factor is vascularity. Blanching on pressure and the presence of dermal bleeding are both evidence of an active circulation. When there is some doubt the anatomy of the region together with the size and content of the pedicle help in making a decision (Fig. 1.6). The problem arises most acutely in the face and scalp and there the vascular abundance is on the side of survival, and

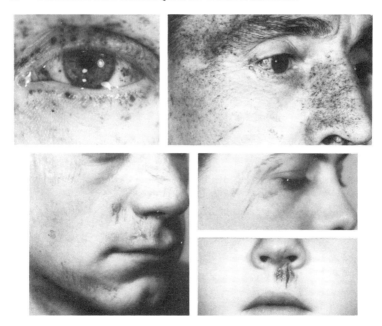

Fig. 1.3 Examples of tattooed scarring resulting from failure to remove ingrained dirt and grit from the wound at the time of the injury. At this late stage such tattooing is virtually impossible to eradicate completely.

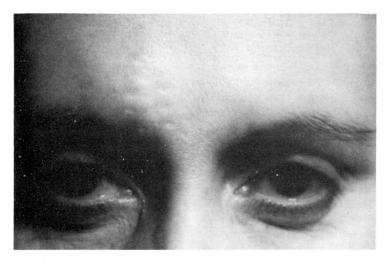

Fig. 1.4 Cross-hatched suture marks caused by coarse sutures left in for too long. Such scarring is difficult or impossible to remove completely.

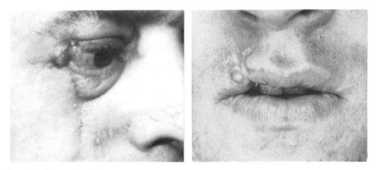

Fig. 1.5 Examples of irregularities of eyelid and mouth resulting from failure to suture matching points together accurately.

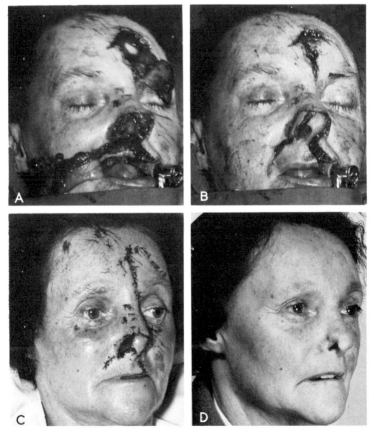

Fig. 1.6 Example of survival and non-survival of traumatic flaps in the face, treated conservatively.

A and B   Flaps before suture showing extent of injury.
    C   Survival and non-survival of flaps.
    D   Late result prior to reconstruction of ala of nose.

flaps should not lightly be excised. In the scalp a flap with any attachment at all should be conserved.

The state of vascularity in general and not merely viability of tissue is significant in almost all aspects of plastic surgery and skin colour consequently requires to be assessed frequently and accurately. For this reason the antiseptic chosen for skin sterilisation should be one which does not stain the skin or tissues. Merthiolate and iodine, suitable otherwise, should not be used; satisfactory agents are cetrimide and chlorhexidine ('Hibitane').

In preparing a wound for suture the wound edge should be vertical if the best scar result is to be achieved and as a corollary of this surgical incisions must also be made vertical. Accurate suturing is also very much easier when the faces of tissue brought together are of the same thickness. If the wound is being sutured without tension all that may be required to prepare the skin edges is to undercut each edge for 3 to 6 mm to allow slight wound eversion.

When there is tension steps can be taken in preparing the wound to eliminate it or at least prevent its worst consequences by undercutting or the use of the Z-plasty.

Undercutting (Fig. 1.7). This allows a degree of advancement of the skin. In undercutting, level is important and depends on the vascularity of the flaps and on the depth of important nerves. In the face the appropriate level is just deep to the dermis, for any undercutting must be superficial to the level of the branches of the facial nerve. The blood supply of facial skin is excellent and necrosis is unlikely to follow undercutting at even such a superficial level. In the scalp the plane between galea aponeurotica and pericranium is used and multiple relaxation incisions in the deep surface of the galea aponeurotica give a little added advancement. In the limbs and trunk it is wiser if undercutting has to be more than minimal to use the plane of cleavage between superficial and deep fascia.

Surgeons vary greatly in the extent to which they use undercutting in wound preparation. To avoid more than minimal undercutting wherever possible reduces enormously the chance of haematoma since there is nowhere for it to collect.

Z-plasty. The use of the Z-plasty in this situation will be discussed in chapter 2. When the method is employed it is naturally used in conjunction with undercutting.

If it is clear that even with maximal undercutting closure will not be achieved the usual procedure especially in the case of a traumatic wound is to use a free skin graft. On occasion a more complicated flap procedure may be feasible but it is seldom a good method for emergency use. The free skin graft is safer and simpler.

FACE

LIMBS &
TRUNK

SCALP

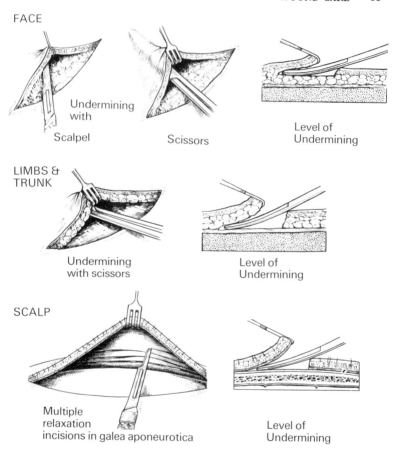

Undermining
with
Scalpel   Scissors

Level of
Undermining

Undermining
with scissors

Level of
Undermining

Multiple
relaxation
incisions in galea aponeurotica

Level of
Undermining

Fig. 1.7 The methods and levels of undermining in the face, limbs and trunk, and scalp.

STITCHCRAFT

When the surgeon is aiming to make his scar as inconspicuous as possible suturing of the wound becomes an extremely precise procedure and good results cannot be expected unless the suture materials, the needles and the instruments are suitable.

SUTURE MATERIALS

The preferences of surgeons play a large part in their personal selection of suture materials. At the same time different materials vary in their properties and these properties determine which particular material is the appropriate one in a given situation. The commonly used threads are:

Braided silk
This material, judged on its handling and knotting characteristics, provides the ideal against which other suture materials are matched. It is normally supplied waterproofed and this is said to reduce reaction around the suture holes. Its major defect is the fact that despite waterproofing it tends to give rise to more tissue reaction than synthetic materials though whether this is sufficient to make any difference to the ultimate scar in the long term is doubtful. Its tensile strength though less than that of the synthetics is nonetheless more than adequate for most purposes.

Synthetics
Examples of these are braided nylon, braided polyester fibre, polythene and monofilament nylon. The main virtues claimed for them are improvement in tensile strength and reduction in tissue reaction. Generally their acceptability depends on how nearly they handle like silk. The recent braided products are more successful in this respect and in most cases their usefulness is a matter of personal preference. The reduction in tissue reaction due to epithelial down-growth along the track of the suture is useful when skin sutures are being left for more than the usual period as sometimes in hand surgery. The monofilament sutures tend to have unsatisfactory knotting properties because of the smoothness of their surface though some surgeons accept this because they feel that the lack of tissue reaction more than compensates. The smooth surface is a definite advantage when the material is used as a continuous intradermal suture since it makes removal easy.

Catgut
To help relieve tension catgut has been recommended as a buried suture. Its use is discussed on page 21.

NEEDLES

Atraumatic sutures are now universal and the problem of needles which can be used with the Gillies needle holder has been solved with the introduction by Messrs. Ethicon of their 'slim-line needle' range of sutures. Other manufacturers are now somewhat belatedly also supplying sutures with comparable needles.

INSTRUMENTS (Fig. 1.8)

The instruments concerned are *needle-holders, dissecting forceps, skin hooks* and *scissors*.

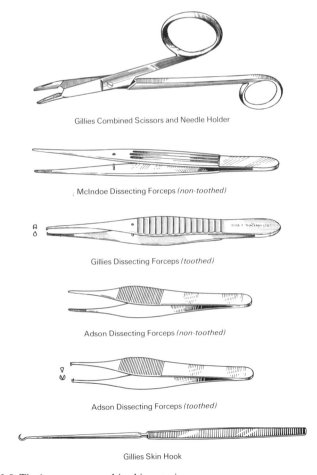

Gillies Combined Scissors and Needle Holder

McIndoe Dissecting Forceps *(non-toothed)*

Gillies Dissecting Forceps *(toothed)*

Adson Dissecting Forceps *(non-toothed)*

Adson Dissecting Forceps *(toothed)*

Gillies Skin Hook

Fig. 1.8 The instruments used in skin suturing.

It is preferable to use the instrumental method of suture tying (Fig. 1.9) for the small needles and fine suture materials make tying by hand clumsy and difficult. With instrumental tying tension can be regulated and knot placement carried out with much greater finesse, exactitude and expedition after only a little practice. The needle-holders normally used in general surgery are quite useless. Large, cumbersome and ill-designed for the necessarily fine work of careful skin suturing, the locking mechanism in particular makes them impossible to use for knot tying. The Gillies needle-holder or one of its modifications is essential. Though it takes a little time to acquire skill in its use it is a most rewarding facility to possess. The needle is usually held transversely in its jaws but the instrument is

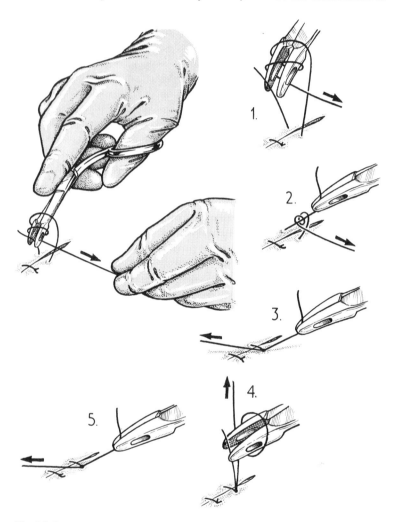

Fig. 1.9 Instrumental tying of a suture.

constructed so that it is possible also to hold the needle lengthwise rigidly (Fig. 1.10). This can be quite an advantage in a difficult situation, particularly when a fully curved needle is being used.

The more a wound edge is traumatised the less good will be the cosmetic result and so the implements for holding wound margins steady for suturing must be as atraumatic as possible. The skin hook is the least traumatic instrument though its method of use, described below, is a difficult one to use with elegance and speed. Because of this dissecting forceps are more routinely used; individual preference will decide the choice of the toothed or non-toothed varieties,

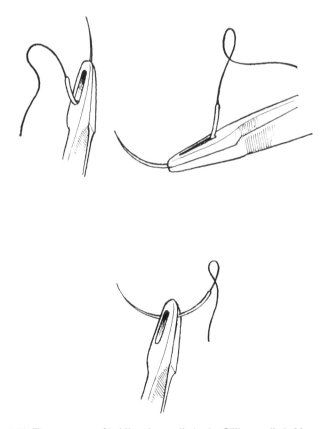

Fig. 1.10 The two ways of holding the needle in the Gillies needle holder.

but both should be used with due regard to the trauma they are causing. The McIndoe and Gillies dissecting forceps are of a suitable size for routine suturing but for really fine work Adson forceps are preferable.

Two types of scissors are usually employed, straight sharp-pointed for cutting wound margins and suture removal, curved blunt-pointed for undercutting wound edges. Both should be sharp so that tissues are cut cleanly and not crushed.

TECHNIQUE OF WOUND SUTURE

The aim is to produce an absolutely accurately coapted wound atraumatically and technique of handling and suturing is merely a means to this end. First time accurate placing of the suture is a habit to acquire, the second attempt is all too often worse than the first and only results in a moth-eaten wound edge and poor scar.

The surgeon must, as far as possible, be in a comfortable relaxed position with elbows braced against the body or otherwise supported so that movement is largely confined to wrist and fingers. The steadiness of such a posture permits much more smooth and precise movements.

The needle is curved and so moves most readily in a circle. The wrist must therefore be brought freely into play so that insertion and pull through of the needle are in the line of its curve (Fig. 1.11).

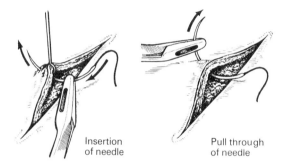

Insertion
of needle

Pull through
of needle

Fig. 1.11 The insertion and pull through of a needle in the line of the curve of the needle.

For a definite period after a wound is sutured slight oedema of the wound tends to develop and though it can be reduced by a pressure dressing, allowance must be made for it in tying the suture. If the suture is too tight it will surely cut in more rapidly and make a suture mark. The correct suture tension just avoids blanching the skin held by the suture.

Sutures may be **interrupted** or **continuous**. When the cosmetic result is all important the interrupted suture is best but the continuous is often adequate in other circumstances, e.g. delay of flap or pedicle.

Interrupted sutures

The usual suture is the **simple loop suture** (Fig. 1.12) which consists of a simple loop knotted at one or other side of the wound. It aims to bring the skin edges together absolutely accurately with no overlapping of one margin. A general tendency towards slight 'pouting' of the suture line helps to ensure complete dermal apposition and makes sure that inversion of the wound edges is avoided. Inverted wound edges heal more slowly and give a poorer scar. In addition the inverted scar creates a shadow which draws attention to it, detracting further from its appearance. A shadow similarly tends to occur when edge to edge opposition is not accurate. It is to allow the desired degree of eversion that a skin edge is sometimes undermined for 3 to 6 mm.

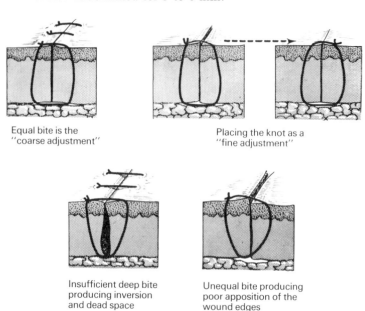

Equal bite is the "coarse adjustment"

Placing the knot as a "fine adjustment"

Insufficient deep bite producing inversion and dead space

Unequal bite producing poor apposition of the wound edges

Fig. 1.12 The simple loop suture.

The suture should include at least the whole dermis and the needle should take an equal bite of each side. The taking of an equal bite might be termed 'coarse adjustment' of getting the wound edges level. Not infrequently, however, one or other edge is a shade higher than its fellow and the lower side can be raised a little by manipulating the knot in tying to that side of the wound. Every suture has an optimal side for its knot and its manipulation is the 'fine adjustment'.

By making the suture take a slightly greater bite of the deeper part, dermis or fat, the whole face of wound margin is approximated and the very slight eversion achieved. When a curved needle is used the wound edge is held everted (Fig. 1.13) and the needle directed so

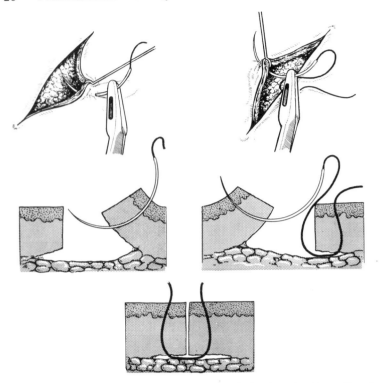

Fig. 1.13 Everting the wound edge with a skin hook before inserting the needle and the path of the curved needle in the skin.

that its path will make a curve in the appropriate direction when the skin is allowed to fall back into its normal position. This eversion is carried out with the least trauma when a skin hook is used. It is technically much easier as a rule to suture from the more mobile side of the wound to the more fixed side. The side of the thumb can also be used to evert the skin during insertion of sutures (Fig. 1.14).

Where the skin is thin and poorly supported or mobile on its deep surface, e.g. around the eyelids, it is particularly difficult to avoid inversion and the best solution is often to use the *vertical mattress suture* (Fig. 1.15). This suture has no greater tendency to leave stitch marks than any other if the sutures are not tied too tightly and are removed early, and if the superficial bite is minimal the tendency to invert is corrected.

When there is no tension of the wound the interrupted suture alone is adequate. When there is tension two possible additional measures are described which are said to allow early removal of skin

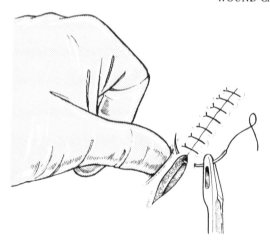

Fig. 1.14 The use of the thumb to evert the skin during the insertion of a suture.

sutures without wound disruption or stretching, namely the use of buried catgut sutures or a continuous intradermal suture.

Buried catgut sutures (Fig. 1.15). Interrupted buried catgut sutures with the knot placed deeply are used with the idea of taking strain after early removal of skin sutures. Their ability to prevent wound stretching is rather doubtful; the result is usually as good or bad as might have been expected had they not been used. Their main value is probably to eliminate dead space and prevent haematoma.

Continuous intradermal suture (Fig. 1.15). This suture has the merit that it can be left in for 10 to 12 days without leaving suture marks. Though it may be used by itself it will be found that really accurate skin edge apposition is only possible if additional interrupted skin sutures are used. Its role then is to take any tension from the interrupted sutures. Monofilament nylon can be used.

While these methods are used and recommended in textbooks their value is very limited and the Z-plasty used in conjunction with extensive undercutting is more effective. If these are not practicable or cannot be employed to the full some degree of stretching is probably inevitable.

Continuous sutures

The most useful continuous sutures are the **'blanket stitch'** and the **continuous 'over and over'** (Fig. 1.15). The 'blanket stitch' has the advantage of not 'bunching up' the wound and a double turn at each stitch converts it into a locked suture. The 'over and over' suture unfortunately does tend to bunch the wound. Naturally such sutures cannot be placed quite as accurately as the interrupted suture but where an impeccable scar is not essential they certainly save time. It is sometimes stated that the continuous suture tends to strangulate the wound edge but this is due to unduly tight insertion rather than any inherent defect of the method.

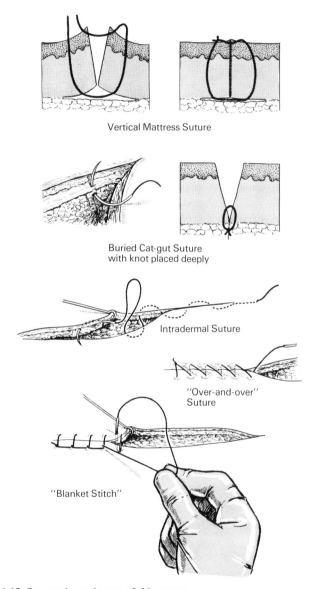

Vertical Mattress Suture

Buried Cat-gut Suture
with knot placed deeply

Intradermal Suture

"Over-and-over"
Suture

"Blanket Stitch"

Fig. 1.15 Commonly used types of skin suture.

DISTRIBUTION OF WOUND TENSION

When a wound is tending to distort and it is difficult to distribute the tension evenly on both sides for suturing it often helps to make the wound taut with a skin hook in each end so that a few key sutures can be placed accurately before inserting the intervening sutures. When distortion is to be expected and especially in a curved incision trouble will be saved by tattooing matching points (Fig. 1.16) with Bonney's Blue* (Pig. Tinctorium, B.P.C.) on either side of the projected incision before any cut is made.

THE THREE-POINT SUTURE (Fig. 1.17)

Where a triangular flap has to be inset it is often difficult to get the tip of the flap to lie in position, yet multiple sutures placed through the full thickness of the dermis are apt to strangulate the tissue at the tip and produce necrosis. The three-point suture in such a situation helps to avoid necrosis while holding the tip in place. As frequently

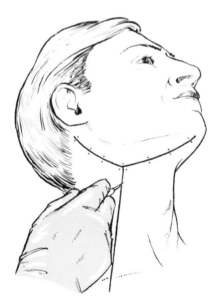

Fig. 1.16 The three-point suture.

* Bonney's Blue:

Gentian Violet	10 g
Brilliant Green	10 g
Alcohol (95%)	950 ml
Water to	2000 ml

described the suture tends to bunch the tip of the flap and a minor variation is recommended which is theoretically sound and effective in practice in holding the tip without bunching. The points to be noted in inserting the suture are:

1. To make sure that the suture leaves and enters the reception side of the wound at the same level as its placement in the V flap.

2. To make the suture emerge well back on the reception side of the wound.

The principle of the three-point suture can be extended for use where two flaps are being approximated to the third side of a wound.

LENGTH OF SCAR AND THE 'DOG-EAR'

When an oval or circular lesion is excised and the defect closed by direct suture the resulting scar is always considerably longer than the original lesion, a fact which it is always wise to explain to the patient.

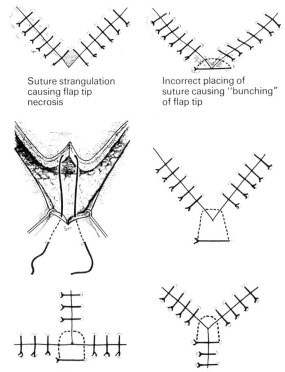

Suture strangulation causing flap tip necrosis

Incorrect placing of suture causing "bunching" of flap tip

Method of insertion and applications of the three point suture

Fig. 1.17 The three-point suture.

This is so for two reasons:

1. When the curved lines, ellipse up to circle, resulting from the excision are brought together in a straight line the result naturally is lengthening of the scar.

2. When the ellipse following excision is sutured there is almost invariably at each end of the suture line a 'dog-ear' and the correction of this lengthens the scar still further.

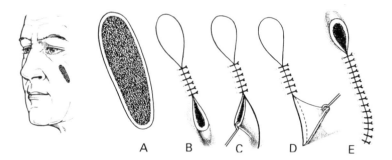

A   B   C   D   E

Fig. 1.18 Removal of a 'dog-ear'. Following excision of the lesion (A), the skin defect is sutured (B) until the 'dog-ear' becomes apparent. The 'dog-ear' is defined with a skin hook and the skin is incised (C) round the base. Excess skin is defined and removed (D), and the skin is sutured (E).

To remove a dog-ear (Fig. 1.18) the wound should be sutured until the elevation becomes pronounced. A hook placed in the end of the wound and raised defines the extent of the dog-ear. The elevation is then excised by incising around the base on one or other side ending up in the line of the wound. The resulting flap is brought across the wound so that the excess skin can be defined and removed. The resulting line has a slight curve and its direction,

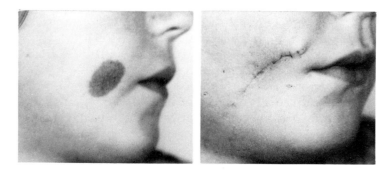

Fig. 1.19 The result of failure to excise a 'dog-ear'.

which depends on the side of the dog-ear cut initially, can be chosen to fit the best line cosmetically. Failure to remove the dog-ear leaves a rather unsightly swelling (Fig. 1.19) and though it flattens somewhat with the passage of time if does tend to remain prominent enough to mar an otherwise satisfactory result.

HAEMATOMA

Where a wound has been sutured, whether it be incision, laceration, flap transfer, etc., the most important single factor causing complications and bad results where surgery had otherwise been soundly planned and adequately carried out is **haematoma**. It acts disastrously in several ways.

Firstly, it raises the general tension of the wound and acts as a foreign body which has either to be evacuated or organised, frequently leading in any case to excessive fibrosis and scar tissue formation. Secondly, it provides a very excellent culture medium for organisms which in its absence would merely be commensals and is readily converted into a collection of pus. Thirdly, in the case of flap transfers it prevents the rapid vascular link-up (p. 119) between raw surfaces which is an essential part of these procedures. In grafting too it plays an important role in graft failure though this aspect is discussed in detail later (p. 61).

It is generally true that in a wound with an adequate blood supply and no obvious source of contamination the occurrence of infection can nearly always be traced to haematoma. Indeed it is remarkable just how much contamination a wound can tolerate without clinical sepsis where there is no haematoma.

Even with the greatest care it is not always possible to avoid haematoma however and the problem of treatment then arises. One's natural instinct is to evacuate the clot as soon as it is diagnosed but while early evacuation is sometimes effective the bleeding which gave rise to the original haematoma is very apt to begin again and cause recurrence. In addition the suture line has to be opened enough to allow extrusion of the haematoma and the handling, pressure, etc., needed to squeeze out the fairly solid clot has an unfortunate habit of causing further wound dehiscence.

A valuable alternative method of managing the situation is to await natural liquefaction of the clot, which usually takes about 10 days, and then aspirate through a wide bore needle inserted obliquely at a distance from the suture line. At this stage there is no tendency to fresh bleeding and recurrence of the condition. The problem in the interval is infection and here antibiotics have a useful if limited place. Once infection develops evacuation by opening the suture line or even incision and drainage may be needed though spontaneous discharge may occur. With a low-grade infection aspiration may suffice if the clot *cum* pus has become sufficiently fluid.

It is very much a condition where prevention is better than cure and such measures as can be used to prevent its occurrence— meticulous haematosis, avoidance of dead space, judicious use of pressure dressings, use of drains with or without suction when its occurrence is otherwise considered inevitable—will help to prevent it from playing its usual sinister role in unsatisfactory healing and excessive scar formation.

POSTOPERATIVE CARE

The aim of good postoperative treatment is to **prevent haematoma, provide rest for healing** and **prevent suture marks**. In practice this is achieved by the dressing, care in suture removal and later support of the wound.

The dressing
With extensive undermining it is difficult despite meticulous haemostasis to prevent a haematoma unless steps are taken to prevent it.

In the past, the pressure dressing was the means usually employed, used with or without a drain. The pressure dressing apart from preventing haematoma provided the immobility and splinting which creates the best conditions for rapid, uneventful healing and controls the oedema which begins the cutting in process of a suture. More recently suction drainage has tended to replace it in its role of preventing haematoma. It can often be used with the wound exposed and this may be regarded as an advantage in certain circumstances. On occasion the two may be combined to good effect, the suction being removed when drainage stops, leaving the pressure dressing to be removed when the sutures are due for removal.

In the face where there has been minimal undermining, particularly around the mouth, the advantages of a pressure dressing may be more than outweighed by the almost inevitable contamination with food and saliva and it is often found that exposure of the wound gives a better result. It is then essential to keep the suture line dry and free of blood clot until the fibrin clot covering the line of the wound is firm and dry.

The wide mesh of a *single layer* of tulle gras allows the passage of any discharge and this combined with the vaseline base make it a particularly good dressing next the wound as it permits the dressing to be removed with the minimum of trauma from sticking. Over the tulle gras, gauze and wool followed by a crepe bandage will give adequate, cushioned pressure and immobility. Elastoplast may replace the crepe bandage in suitable circumstances and the adhesive properties of the elastoplast can be greatly enhanced by preliminary painting of the skin with Mastisol.

An alternative dressing applied directly to the suture line is 'micropore' skin tape. Used in this way it has characteristics which are extremely convenient. It does not macerate the skin, it supports the wound well and yet, peeled off slowly, sticks neither to suture or hair. Apart from its role in the sutured wound, it can also on occasion be used to coapt wound edges and obviate the need for sutures at all, a considerable virtue when the young child with a laceration is being treated.

Applied directly over the wound its adhesiveness encourages the wound edges to lie flush, a useful attribute when flap tips are tending to lie a little proud of the wound as a whole.

If no undermining has been used, such tape can provide the sole dressing but equally a pressure dressing can be applied over it.

Suture removal
It is usual to lay down set days for the removal of sutures in various sites and under varying circumstances but this is quite a wrong approach. Clinical experience soon tells the surgeon when a suture may safely be removed. Naturally the principle is to remove at the earliest time judged safe and this depends on so many factors, degree of tension, site, line of wound, etc., that it is quite impossible to lay down rules. In actually removing the suture (Fig. 1.20) one must remember that the tensile strength of the wound is minimal and dehiscence is liable to occur on the slightest provocation. Where most care is needed the sutures are usually smallest and therefore before beginning there must be a good light, fine, sharp scissors which cut to the point and fine dissecting forceps which grip properly. With these prerequisites the actual technique of removal is not radically different from ordinary suture removal except that absolute gentleness is necessary and the cut suture being pulled out must always be pulled out towards the wound.

Scissors of course are not invariably sharp and do not always cut to the point and a good alternative method is to use the tip of a triangular scalpel blade (Fig. 1.20) to cut the suture. In a difficult

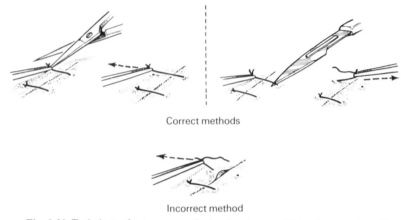

Correct methods

Incorrect method

Fig. 1.20 Technique of suture removal, showing the use of iris scissors and no. 11 scalpel blade. Correctly removed, the suture is pulled *towards* the wound; incorrect removal, pulling the suture away from the wound, causes added tension and may even disrupt the wound.

situation its extremely sharp fine point will often cut the suture with much less disturbance of the wound than scissors.

In removal as in insertion of the suture the surgeon should support his elbows and work from wrist and fingers to give smooth movements without tremor. The patient equally should be carefully supported so that the suture line stays absolutely still.

Subsequent support of the wound
As already stated, early suture removal leaves a wound devoid of strength so that a sudden ill-judged tension strain may cause it to open. For this reason the wound is best supported or at least protected up to a week after stitch removal and micropore skin tape works well in this role. It is seldom practicable to support the wound much beyond this and indeed attempts to prevent later stretching of the wound by prolonged support are of little avail.

KELOIDS AND HYPERTROPHIC SCARS

When a scar, instead of becoming soft and pale in the usual manner, becomes red and thickened it is described as being either a hypertrophic scar or a keloid.

These terms tend to be used rather indiscriminately, probably because it is difficult to define each with certainty. The typical hypertrophic scar is raised, rather red initially, but does not encroach on the surrounding normal skin, does not give rise to symptoms, and shows an eventual tendency to regress. The keloid tends to be a much more florid lesion; it is grossly elevated, tends to spread and involve the surrounding normal skin, and gives rise to symptoms of itching, a feeling of hotness, and tenderness to touch.

These are the extremes and as such easily recognised but in reality there is an infinite graduation from the completely quiescent scar through the very mildly hypertrophic scar to the most severe of keloids and the point at which a hypertrophic scar becomes a keloid is a matter of opinion. The name is fortunately of subsidiary importance for the treatment of both conditions is similar. Indeed the gradation rather suggests that the arbitrary division into keloid and hypertrophic scar is artificial and that the conditions are really a single entity of varying severity. Virtually nothing is known of the cause.

The clinical picture
A precise picture is difficult to draw, for clinical generalisations do not necessarily apply to the individual case and the condition itself is extremely variable and unpredictable. In the description which follows the term keloid will be used to cover both conditions.

The tendency to develop keloids diminishes greatly with age but it is not possible in practice to forecast whether any particular patient will develop a keloid. Nevertheless, any incision in a known 'keloid former' is more likely to develop into a keloid than a similar incision in a random patient and recurrence following simple excision of a keloid is highly probable. Keloids are undoubtedly much more common in the negro than in the white patient. The negro also exhibits the condition in its most active form and the 'tumours' can on occasion reach quite grotesque proportions. In the white on the other hand even the frank keloid does eventually become less active and takes on the characters and activity rather of a hypertrophic scar (Fig. 1.21).

Certain areas of the body have a particular tendency to produce keloids (Fig. 1.22); the presternal area is probably the most prone of all and here oddly enough the shape of the keloid often shows a sex difference—in the male it tends to be irregular in outline, in the female the pull of the breasts commonly gives it a butterfly outline. The deltoid area is another notorious site. It is significant that a scar may become keloid in only part of its length and this shows particularly in the neck where the vertical scar is very subject to keloid change while the horizontal scar is seldom affected. This indeed is one of the facts which the various theories of causation fail to explain for if a scar of neck is excised incorporating Z-plasties it is not uncommon for the horizontal scars to be completely flat and soft while the vertical limbs of the Zs show keloid or at very least hypertrophic change. In general, scars in lines or election show less tendency to keloid than those which cross them.

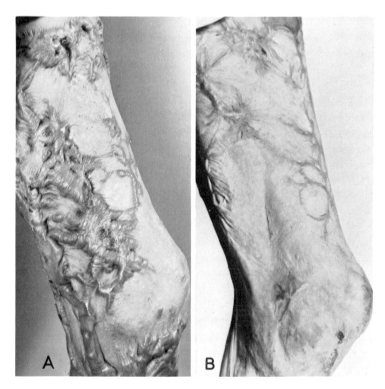

Fig. 1.21 Change from keloid to hypertrophic scarring over a period of two years.

Treatment
Prior to the introduction of the highly active local steroid, triamcinolone, the mainstay of treatment was X-ray therapy. Whether or not the method had any real value or whether it was merely being given credit for the spontaneous tendency to regression is difficult to tell. It did reduce the associated itch but with the advent of triamcinolone it has little place in therapy. Certainly its use should never be countenanced in the young patient with a life-time ahead of him and as the major problem in practice is the child with extensive post-burn keloid, the uselessness of X-ray therapy needs no emphasis. In the young child with keloid it is probably wise to restrict therapy to control of the itch and await spontaneous regression. For this purpose local steroid applied as an ointment usually works well.

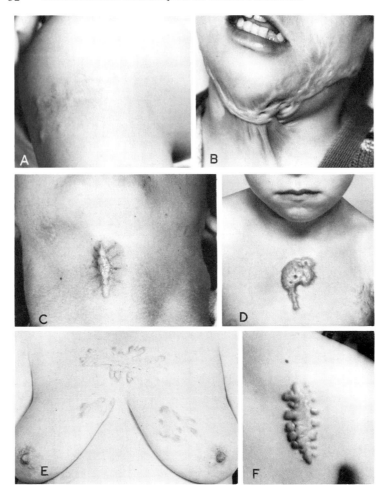

Fig. 1.22 Examples of keloids and hypertrophic scars.
A   Mildly hypertrophic scar of deltoid region.
B   Severe postburn hypertrophic scarring of neck and chin.
C   Hypertrophic scarring following the ill-judged use of a vertical incision to excise a thyroglossal fistula.
D   Presternal keloid in the male.
E   Presternal keloid in the female, showing butterfly outline.
F   Severe keloid of scapular region.

The circumscribed keloid might appear to be more of a candidate for X-ray therapy but it is in this type of keloid that triamcinolone injected into its substance is most dramatically successful, with obvious flattening and softening in a matter of days. It must nevertheless be remembered always that triamcinolone is itself an extremely potent drug whose action locally is not fully understood.

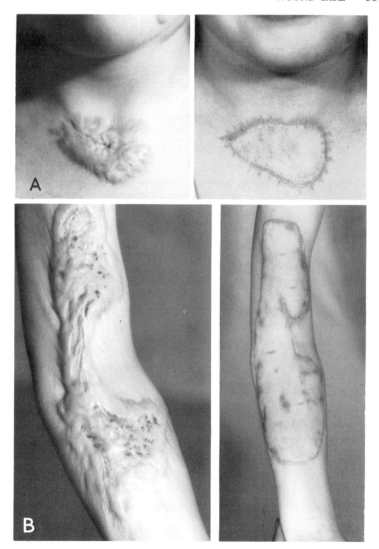

Fig. 1.23 Marginal recurrence of keloid after excision and grafting.

Caution in its use is thus absolutely essential. It must be injected actually into the substance of the keloid and enough is injected to make the whole keloid blanch. Injection can be repeated weekly. When the keloid has become flat with the surrounding skin treatment should stop; further injections will produce local skin and fat atrophy. Remarkably enough the drug is effective regardless of whether the keloid is red and 'fresh' or white and 'mature'.

Where in the past it was usual to give prophylactic X-ray therapy if keloid was expected after surgery it is probably safe enough now to wait and treat with triamcinolone at the first sign of trouble. In the worst sites, nevertheless, particularly the presternal area, surgery of any kind should be contemplated with extreme reluctance. A bigger keloid is the most likely result (Fig. 1.23).

With the greatest care and the best treatment the results still leave a good deal to be desired. One's impression is that the process is dampened down rather than stopped completely and the extent to which it is reduced depends on its inherent activity. At one end of the scale mild hypertrophy can be stopped completely while at the other the florid keloid in a bad site is less effectively controlled. Fortunately, the condition is commoner in its less active form and time is always on the side of regression and resolution.

2

The Z-plasty

The Z-plasty is a procedure which involves the transposition of two interdigitating triangular flaps. Its name derives from the fact that, drawn out on the skin, the three limbs of the flaps have the overall shape of a Z. Although hallowed by long usage the name is not strictly accurate since the limbs are equal in length.

Transposition of the flaps has several effects (Fig. 2.1) of which two have special relevance:

1. There is a gain in length along the direction of the common limb of the Z.

2. The common limb of the Z becomes changed in direction.

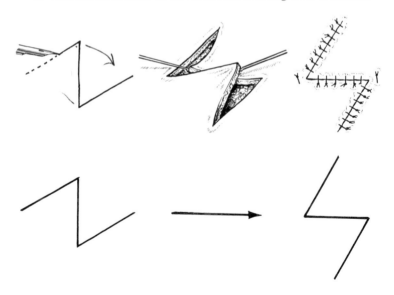

Fig. 2.1 The Z-plasty.

It is exploitation of these effects which makes the Z-plasty one of the most useful as well as one of the most widely used procedures in plastic surgery. Its worth has been established in two sets of circumstances, the **treatment of contractures** when we make use of the phenomenon of lengthening, and the **management of facial scars** when we make use of the fact that the common limb changes in direction. Although both lengthening and change of direction occur together it is usually only one of the two aspects which concerns the surgeon at any particular time. The simultaneous and inescapable accomplishment of the other is usually a bonus but it can be a nuisance.

USE IN CONTRACTURES

The basic manoeuvre
When the Z-plasty is used in a contracture the common limb, i.e. the central limb of the Z, lies along the line of the contracture to be released. The usual size of each of the angles of the Z is 60°, a compromise figure which has been reached as a result of experience. The reasons for selecting this angle size and the effects of altering it will be discussed later but 60° will be the size used in the present discussion.

Constructed in this way the two triangles together have the shape of a parallelogram with its shorter diagonal in the line of the contracture, its longer diagonal perpendicular to it. The two diagonals can conveniently be referred to as the **contractural diagonal** and the **transverse diagonal** (Fig. 2.2).

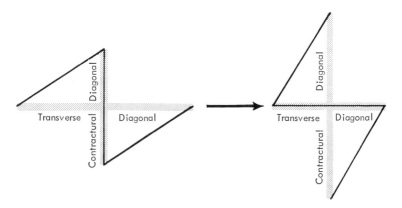

Fig. 2.2 The diagonals of the Z-plasty, showing how the contractural diagonal lengthens and the transverse diagonal shortens correspondingly.

To understand the sequence of events when a Z-plasty is used in a contracture it is essential to bear in mind that the common limb of the Z, being along the line of the contracture, is under considerable tension. Because of this its ends spring apart as the fibrous tissue band along the contracture line is divided when the flaps are raised. Springing apart of the divided contracture has the effect of changing the shape of the parallelogram and causes the triangular flaps to become transposed, the contractural diagonal to lengthen and the transverse diagonal to shorten (Fig. 2.3).

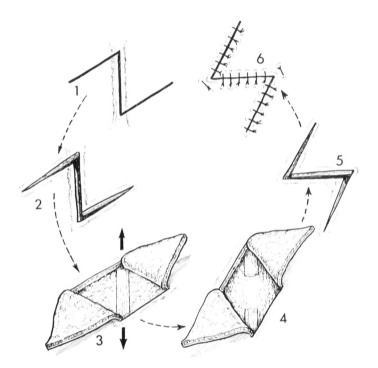

Fig. 2.3 A schematic formalised representation of the several stages of the Z-plasty.

It is important to appreciate that the surgeon does not actively transpose the Z flaps when a Z-plasty is used properly to correct a linear contracture; flap transposition follows naturally from the change in shape of the parallelogram.

The changes in length are such that the length of the contractural diagonal *after* transposition equals that of the transverse diagonal *before* transposition. Increase in length of the contractural diagonal has been achieved at the expense of the transverse diagonal which has shortened as much as the contractural diagonal has lengthened.

Translated into practical terms this means that skin has been brought in from the sides with a tightening effect, as shown by the shortening of the transverse diagonal, to achieve the lengthening of the contractural diagonal; the difference in length of the two diagonals indicates the actual amount of lengthening and shortening.

The surgeon is naturally more interested in the lengthening than the shortening which inevitably accompanies it but it is crucial to successful Z-plasty practice to bear in mind that without the transverse shortening there will be no lengthening. In practical terms, unless transverse slack is available to be taken up, equal in quantity to the length difference between the axes of the Z, the method will not work.

Construction of the Z
Since the skin flaps must fit together in their transposed position the limbs of the Z must of necessity be equal in length. The angles of the Z are also usually made equal in size. The factors in construction which do vary are **angle size** and **limb length** and the ways in which these variable factors affect the result provides an explanation of why a specific construction is used in a particular set of circumstances.

Angle size. Once the lengths of the limbs of the Z has been decided the lengthening to be expected depends entirely on the size of the angle and as the angle increases so too does the amount of lengthening. With an angle of 30° there is theoretically a 25 per cent increase in length, with 45° a 50 per cent increase, while with an angle of 60° the increase rises to 75 per cent (Fig. 2.4). It must be stressed that at all times it is *percentage* increase of length which is controlled by size of angle. These increases are theoretical and cannot be applied clinically with strict accuracy, although when account is taken of variations in skin extensibility, presence of scarring, etc., it is

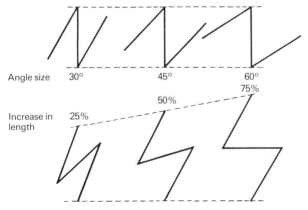

Fig. 2.4 The percentage increase of length which results from the use of different angle sizes.

surprising how well they do apply. The actual lengthening is usually a little less than the theoretical one.

In theory angles of up to and beyond 90° could be used with steady increase in the amount of lengthening but in practice limiting factors emerge which determine the optimal angle.

Reduction of the angle much below 60° would defeat the very object of the Z-plasty since the smaller angle would produce less gain in length. In addition, narrowing of the flap significantly would have a disastrous effect on its blood supply.

Increase of the angle much beyond 60° would increase the amount of lengthening but, as already stressed, this would entail an equal amount of transverse shortening. Tissue for transverse shortening is seldom available in unlimited quantity and as the angle increases beyond 60° the tension produced in the surrounding tissues tends to be so great that the flaps cannot readily be brought into their transposed position.

For these reasons 60° is the compromise figure usually used for angle size.

Limb length. Just as angle size controls percentage increase of length so limb length controls the *actual* increase in length since the increase is a proportion of the original length. A longer initial limb results in a greater increase of length for a particular size of angle. Such an increase in the amount of lengthening naturally increases the tissue brought in from the sides.

The factors which limit maximum and minimum angle size have resulted in the compromise use of 60° as the routine Z-plasty angle and it is length of limb which provides the major variable in practice. Regardless of length of contracture the amount of tissue available on either side determines the practicable limb length—a large amount will permit a large Z, a small amount will correspondingly limit the size of the Z.

The single and the multiple Z

The search for ways of reducing the amount of transverse shortening without significantly affecting the amount of lengthening has led to the development of the **multiple Z-plasty** and its advantages are such that it has virtually replaced the single Z-plasty in many clinical situations.

In the single Z-plasty one large Z extends along virtually the entire length of the contracture; in the multiple Z-plasty the contracture is divided into a number of segments on each of which a small Z is constructed.

The contrast between the two can best be appreciated by using a concrete example. If we construct a single Z which is going to achieve 2 cm of lengthening and at the same time construct a series of four small Zs each equal in size to a quarter of the single Z we can compare them from the point of view of lengthening and shortening (Fig. 2.5).

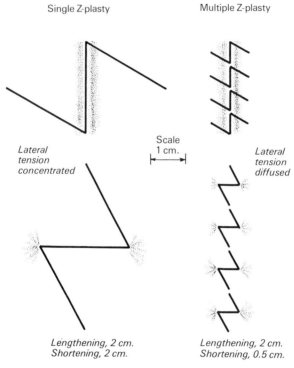

Single Z-plasty

Multiple Z-plasty

Scale
1 cm.

Lateral
tension
concentrated

Lateral
tension
diffused

Lengthening, 2 cm.
Shortening, 2 cm.

Lengthening, 2 cm.
Shortening, 0.5 cm.

Fig. 2.5 Comparison of the lengthening and shortening produced by a single and a multiple Z-plasty. Note also how lateral tension is concentrated by the single Z-plasty and diffused by the multiple Z-plasty.

The single Z achieves 2 cm of lengthening and at the same time there is 2 cm of shortening in the transverse axis.

The multiple Z behaves very differently. Each of the four Zs produces 0·5 cm of lengthening with a corresponding 0·5 cm of shortening at each transverse axis. The lengthening being in series is additive giving an overall lengthening of 2 cm; in contrast the shortening is in parallel and remains 0·5 cm at each Z.

In both the single and multiple Z then the amount of lengthening achieved is the same but the shortening has been greatly reduced by using the multiple Z. Many situations exist in which a Z-plasty could be used to advantage where the tissue cannot stand 2 cm of shortening but could tolerate 0·5 cm with ease. For those the multiple Z-plasty is a possible solution.

The change from single to multiple Z-plasty also alters the type of lateral tension. From being concentrated in the line of the transverse limb of the single Z, it is diffused over the several transverse limbs of the multiple Z-plasty in addition to being reduced, and this has obvious advantages from a vascular point of view.

In the multiple, as in the single Z-plasty, the theoretical lengthening is probably not capable of being achieved for, quite apart from the effect of scarring, etc., there tends to be some loss of lengthening in passage from one Z to the next. Nevertheless the comparison between the two and the advantages of the multiple over the single are still valid.

PRACTICE OF THE Z-PLASTY

From the theoretical discussion it follows that the Z-plasty is most effective where the contracture is narrow and the surrounding tissues are reasonably lax since scarred and contracted tissue on either side can yield no 'slack' to allow lengthening.

This fact explains why the post-burn contracture is so seldom totally correctable by a Z-plasty, single or multiple. The burn scar in contracting has contracted in all directions simultaneously. Although a contracture may be present clinically, skin has really been lost in every axis; the contractural axis is only the most obviously tight. The transverse axis is just as short and unable to shorten any further in the way needed for a successful Z-plasty.

Ideally the central limb of the Z extends the full length of the contracture but this requires a correspondingly large quantity of tissue to be brought in from the sides, tissue which is not always available. It is in the limbs particularly that this problem arises, for such tissue as is available is not concentrated at one point but is spread out along the length of the limb. In such circumstances as have been discussed above the solution may be to construct a series of short Zs instead of one large Z and so bring in from the sides small quantities of tissue all the way down the line of the contracture (Fig. 2.5).

A good measure of the planning and execution of a Z-plasty is the behaviour of the flaps when the contracture is released. If the manoeuvre is indicated and well-planned the flaps should literally fall into their new transposed position; indeed it should be difficult to get them back into their old relationship.

It is when the contracture is of the bowstring type that the Z-plasty is most effective. With the contracture more diffuse in breadth and length it is less satisfactory and a stage is reached where it must be decided whether a Z-plasty is an adequate procedure or whether fresh skin must be imported from elsewhere as a free skin graft. The answer is usually to be found in the surrounding skin; skin must be present as slack at the sides if the contracture is to be released and if it is not obviously available there (Fig. 2.6) the Z-plasty will fail and a free skin graft is the true answer to the problem.

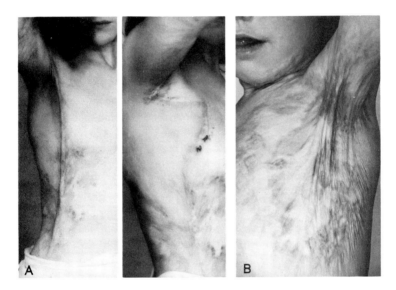

Fig. 2.6 A narrow axillary contracture (A), which is suitable for correction by a Z-plasty, and a diffuse axillary contracture (B), which is unsuitable for a Z-plasty and which requires for its correction the insertion of a split-skin graft.

Planning the Z-plasty (Fig. 2.7 and 2.9)

It may be difficult in planning the procedure to decide where the flaps should be. A good method is to draw an equilateral triangle on each side of the contracture (see Fig. 8.6) and from the resulting parallelogram to select the more suitable of the two sets of limbs. One set may have no particular advantage in which case either may be used. Factors which might favour one set rather than the other are:

1. The flap with the better blood supply is preferable; in particular one with scarring across the base should be avoided.

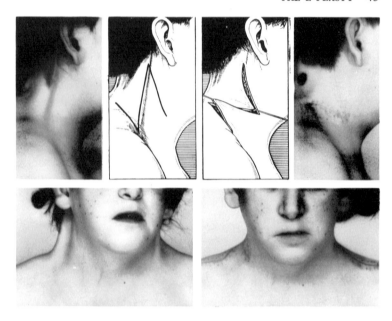

Fig. 2.7 The planning and execution of a *single* Z-plasty to correct the neck webbing componenent of Turner's syndrome.

2. One or other flap may give a scar which will fall into a better line cosmetically. The factors which would influence the choice in such circumstances have already been discussed in Chapter 1.

3. The lie of the flaps and the surrounding skin may permit one set of flaps to rotate more readily into their transposed position.

Skin which is scarred has lost much of its normal elasticity and this may affect slightly the planning of the flaps. A flap of scarred skin should be made a little longer initially than its fellow of normal skin, otherwise the scarred flap will be found to be too short when it is sutured to the unscarred flap.

It is usual though not absolutely essential to have the two angles of equal size. On occasion a line of scarring will limit the angle of one flap and dissimilar angles may then have to be used. Lengthening in such a case becomes the average of the amount to be expected from each angle alone. Indeed if the full quadrilateral of any Z is drawn complete with contractural and transverse diagonals the transverse diagonal will indicate the actual length to be expected when the flaps are transposed.

The multiple Z-plasty

When a single large Z-plasty cannot be used for any of the reasons already discussed the alternative may be to use a multiple Z-plasty. The line of the contracture is then regarded as a series of contracted segments and on each a small Z is constructed creating a line of separate Zs. Such a construction, though it works perfectly well in practice, has been taken a stage further to produce the **continuous multiple Z-plasty** (Fig. 2.8) where the Zs, instead of being individual, form a continuous series giving the appearance of a long line

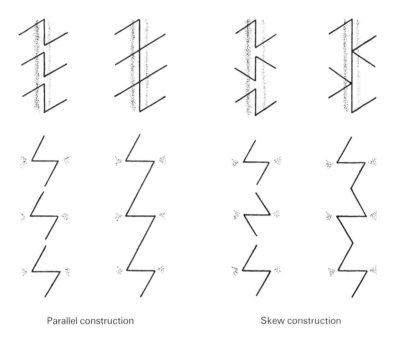

Parallel construction   Skew construction

Fig. 2.8 The evolution of the parallel and skew types of the continuous multiple Z-plasty from a series of interrupted small Z-plasties.

along the contracture with multiple Z side limbs (Fig. 7.8). This is the type of multiple Z-plasty which is now routinely used and it can be constructed with the side limbs either parallel or skew. The presence of scarring in a particular line may influence the construction and make skew flaps preferable but the use of parallel limbs allows the flaps to rotate uniformly in transposition, at the same time preventing the occurrence of the broad tipped flap with its narrow base which is undesirable from a vascular point of view and inevitable with the skew construction.

Whether a multiple Z-plasty must be used will largely depend on the depth of the bowstring. It is unwise to take the side-limbs much beyond the base of the bowstring and if the making of a large Z would encroach on the surrounding flat skin to any extent especially if it tends to be taut, then a multiple Z-plasty (Fig. 2.9) is safer and on the whole just as effective.

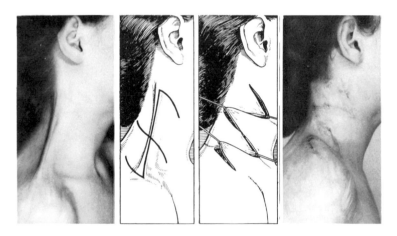

Fig. 2.9 The planning and execution of a *multiple* Z-plasty in correcting a localised postburn contracture of neck.

Blood supply of the flaps

The most frequent complication of the Z-plasty is necrosis of the tip of a flap and it is particularly common if there has been much scarring of the skin. Precautions to avoid necrosis can be taken at all stages of the procedure: by providing the flaps with the maximum of vascular capacity, by avoiding tension and by meticulous haemostasis.

Provision of maximum vascular capacity. This is achieved by designing the flaps broad at the tip, by avoiding scarring across the base and by cutting the flaps as thick as possible. The tip of the flap can be broadened without affecting the angle size by slightly modifying the shape of the flap (Fig. 2.10). The thickest flap practicable should always be cut using the levels of undermining suggested in chapter 1.

Avoidance of undue tension. This can be a very difficult problem particularly when the contracture is a doubtful candidate for Z-plasty or free skin graft. The large, single Z concentrates transverse tension while multiple, small Zs diffuse the tension making it less at

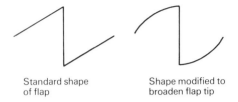

Standard shape
of flap

Shape modified to
broaden flap tip

Fig. 2.10 The modified shape of Z-plasty flap to give maximum vascular capacity.

each individual Z so that embarrassment of the circulation from this cause is reduced to a minimum.

While the contracture may be placed under tension during the procedure to display its line and extent, the parts should be dressed and bandaged in a mid-position to promote relaxation of tissues in all directions.

Meticulous haemostasis. Quite apart from the role it can play in raising flap tension, haematoma predisposes to infection and infection is a potent cause of flap necrosis (p. 119). Careful haemostasis is consequently essential.

USE IN SCARS

It is well recognised that scars in the face tend to be more cosmetically acceptable the more nearly they lie in a line of election; a problem of acceptability is liable to arise when an otherwise satisfactory scar is more than 30° off the line of election. When a Z-plasty is used to improve the appearance of a scar its effect is to break the line of the scar and change its direction. This change takes place with the change in direction of the common limb of the Z. The most desirable result is achieved postoperatively when this common limb is made to lie transversely in a line of election and to this end careful planning is essential.

Siting the Z-plasty

The success of the method used to place the transverse common limb of the completed Z-plasty accurately in terms of size, site and direction depends on two facts. Firstly, if the Z-plasty incisions are made to end on the selected transverse line, transposition of the flaps leaves the transverse common limb automatically lying along the line as planned. Secondly, the limbs of the Z-plasty are equal in length.

If mistakes are to be avoided, the planning of the Z-plasty must be regarded as a formal procedure, to be marked out carefully on the skin before any actual incision is made. The steps themselves are

more easily illustrated than described (Fig. 2.11 and 2.12). With the
scar outlined the line selected for the transverse common limb is
drawn out on the skin with Bonney's Blue, the line naturally being
in a line of election. The length of the intended transverse common
limb, which determines the size of the Z-plasty, is measured out on
the line of the scar, proportioned approximately evenly on each side
of the line selected and drawn out as the transverse common limb.
From each extremity of this measured length a line of equal length is
marked out to meet the line drawn out as the transverse common
limb. This gives three lines of equal length and together they make
the Z-plasty flaps. The fact that the two oblique lines have been
made to end on the selected transverse line means that transposition
of the flaps brings the transverse common limb into the desired line
as planned, and this is true regardless of its direction. Altering its
obliquity merely has the effect of altering the size of the Z-plasty
angle. Increase of obliquity reduces the angle and decrease of
obliquity increases the angle—to a maximum of 60°, at which point
the transverse limb becomes perpendicular to the line of the scar.

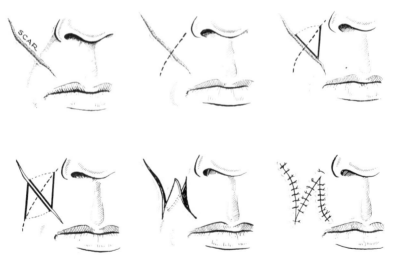

Fig. 2.11 The method of planning a Z-plasty so that the transverse limb of the
completed Z-plasty lies in a predetermined line, in this instance the line of the
nasolabial fold.

As the transverse limb departs from the perpendicular the flap
becomes narrower and the blood supply to its tip increasingly
tenuous. Facial skin with its excellent blood supply is more tolerant of
narrow flaps than skin elsewhere on the body surface but even in the

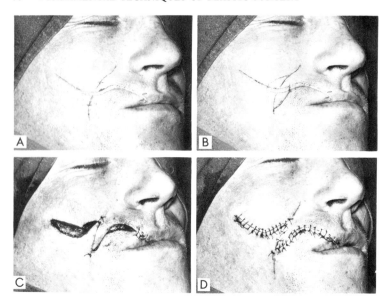

Fig. 2.12 The method illustrated in Figure 2.11 used in practice. A shows the scar outlined and the line of election—the nasolabial fold. B shows the lines of the Z, equal in length with each oblique line ending on the line of election, and C shows the scar excised and the Z flaps transposed. D shows the manoeuvre completed with the transverse limb of the Z lying along the line of election as planned.

face there is a limit to permissible narrowness; a tip angle of 35° is as narrow as can be used with safety. The angle size can fortunately be gauged at the planning stage before any incision is actually made.

Use in facial scars

In the long facial scar it is usual to break the line with more than one Z-plasty and since scars are not invariably straight and lines of election usually run in different directions in different parts of the scar each Z as to be planned strictly on its own. As a rule each will have its individual and quite distinct obliquity. In this way the effect is to convert the single linear scar into a series of smaller scars joined by transverse limbs in lines of election, ideally in actual wrinkle lines. Even at worst, several small scars are usually less conspicuous than the single long scar. It is also found that the large Z-plasty does not give as good a result as the smaller Z. In planning therefore, the estimated length of the transverse limb should be kept fairly small (Fig. 2.13).

When a multiple Z-plasty is used to break up a facial scar problems may result from simultaneous lengthening. A Z-plasty

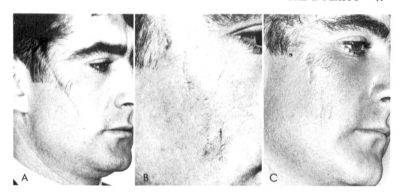

Fig. 2.13 Scar excision with three Z-plasty insets, each with its individually planned transverse limb direction to fit into the local direction of the line of election. A the scar, B early result, C late result.

with the usual angle sizes between 30° and 60° produces a significant amount of lengthening as an automatic and inevitable consequence and this can usually only be accommodated partially without causing distortion which shows as an overlapping of the flaps as they pass from one Z to the next. This overlap is usually excised, in this way reducing the overall lengthening and consequently the greater part of the distortion.

The facial wound which has been sutured under tension is especially prone to stretch and of the various procedures which have been described as helping to prevent stretching the Z-plasty is probably the most valuable where it can be used (Fig. 2.14). Its effect is to break up a long scar with tension directly across the wound into multiple short scars in which tension has been redistributed in such a fashion that the greater part is taken as a shearing strain by each transverse limb of the Z-plasties. It would appear that shearing strains cause much less stretching of the scar than does straight tension. Where the Z-plasty is used for this purpose it is more important to make the transverse limb perpendicular to the general line of the scar than to try and place it in a line of election and the Z-plasty angle should consequently be in the region of 60°.

There are certain further situations in which the Z-plasty acts as an adjunct to other methods designed to minimise scars. In these its effectiveness depends both on the fact of lengthening of the scar and also on accurate placement of its transverse common limb.

The bridle scar

When a scar crosses a hollow, contraction along its line tends to produce a ridged or bridle scar bridging the hollow. In such

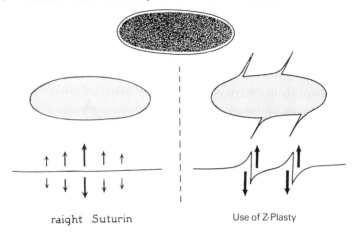

raight Suturin   Use of Z-Plasty

Fig. 2.14 The tension directly across a wound coverted by Z-plasties into a shearing strain taken by the transverse limb of each Z.

circumstances the bridle scar has similarities to a straight contracture and the solution is equally the use of a Z-plasty. This has the effect of lengthening it so that it can sit into the hollow. When the bridle element is short, as in Figure 6.16, a single Z-plasty may be entirely adequate but when the scar is relatively long and bridges a shallow hollow a multiple Z-plasty is more effective (Fig. 2.15).

In the detailed planning of such a multiple Z-plasty there may be the added complication of having to make each transverse limb lie in a line of election to get the best result. So long as it is remembered that it is possible to place each transverse limb independently in such

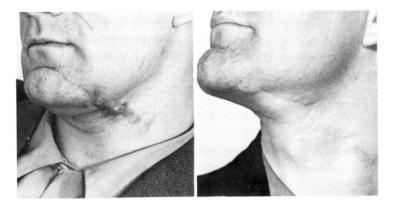

Fig. 2.15 The use of Z-plasties in revising a bridle scar crossing a concavity.

circumstances there should be no difficulty in planning the necessary Z-plasties using the method already described.

The curving scar

This problem is seen in its worst form when a trapdoor of skin lifted, usually as a result of trauma, is merely resutured in place. Contraction of the resulting scar causes elevation of the tissue within its concavity. Seen later it may be assumed, not unreasonably, to be the result of bad suturing but excision of the scar, trimming of the flap quite flat, and resuture with the greatest care only results in recurrence of the original state of affairs within a matter of weeks (Fig. 2.16).

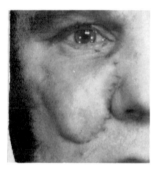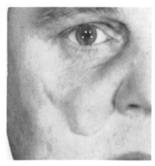

Fig. 2.16 The recurrence of trap-door scarring following simple excision and suture.

Lengthening of the scar by judicious use of the Z-plasty has the effect of preventing recurrence. Here, as in correcting the bridle scar, an effort should be made to place any Z-plasty in a line of election, although with the curving scar the planning of the Z-plasty to give the best result from every point of view can be an extremely difficult exercise and one in which facility comes only with practice (Fig. 2.17).

On occasion the problem of the curving scar takes a slightly different form when the two sides of a wound to be sutured are unequal in length, as in the excision of a 'common-shaped' scar. The taking of unequal bites in suturing can partially equate the lengths but there is a definite limit to this. The Z-plasty can then sometimes help further to reduce the discrepancy in lengths (Fig. 2.18).

The overriding scar

Where there is a tendency to overriding of the tissues on one side

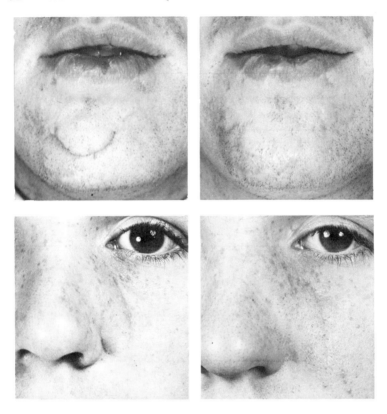

Fig. 2.17 Correction of trap-door scarring following excision and incorporation of Z-plasties.

of a scar the junction between the two sides can usually be smoothed by incorporating one or more Z-plasties when the scar is being excised (Fig. 2.19) and here again the use of lines of election should be remembered.

The decision where and when not to use a Z-plasty in a particular facial scar can be an extremely difficult one in the borderline case, and it is one which must be influenced by the expertise, or its lack, on the part of the surgeon in manipulating the Z-plasty. It can take considerable courage for the inexperienced surgeon to wilfully increase the length of a wound by incorporating one or more Z-plasties, particularly as the early result all too often appears disappointing and only later as the flaps flatten and the scars soften and settle the full benefits become apparent.

A study of how the original scar has behaved is sometimes of help

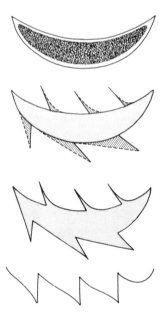

Fig. 2.18 Equalising the lengths of the two sides of a wound previously unequal, by the use of Z-plasties.

in deciding. The scar which has become pale and matches the surrounding skin well is a good candidate, other things being equal. The fully settled scar which has remained conspicuous because it is redder than the surrounding skin, as some scars do even though they have become quite soft, is a bad candidate. The end result is liable merely to be a longer red scar, for each transverse limb stays as red as the rest of the scar and its line fails to fade and merge into the

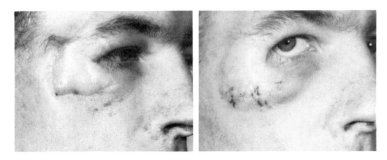

Fig. 2.19 The incorporation of Z-plasties during revision of the scar at the margin of a flap, coupled with thinning of the flap, has the effect of giving a smooth junction between the flap and its surroundings.

background although it is in a line of election. The results of using the Z-plasty in scars tend also to be disappointing in children compared with adults but this is at least partly related to the poor behaviour of scars generally in children, although an added reason is their smooth skin which is able only to lay a scar bare and unable to conceal it in a network of wrinkles. For the same reason the smooth, uncreased adult skin should be viewed with caution.

3

Free skin grafts

As its name implies a free skin graft is completely detached from the body during its transfer from donor to recipient site. From its new habitat it derives a fresh blood supply and develops an attachment. It is used in circumstances which vary enormously and examples of these are:

1. Where there is loss of skin following trauma. Grafting may be carried out **primarily**, immediately after the traumatic episode, or **secondarily**, when granulations have developed.

2. Where a residual skin defect is left following excision of a simple or malignant tumour.

3. Where an ulcer, e.g. gravitational, caused by a non-neoplastic pathological process, is present.

As a general rule a free skin graft will be accepted by any site which, left ungrafted, would rapidly develop granulations. Although most often used to repair a skin defect, such a graft can also cover a defect of the mucosa of the accessible mucous membrane lined cavities—mouth, eye, accessory sinuses, etc.

Free skin grafts (Fig. 3.1) are of two kinds:

1. **Whole skin graft** consisting of epidermis and the full thickness of dermis.

2. **Split-skin graft** consisting of epidermis and a variable quantity of dermis. Split-skin grafts are described as **thin, intermediate** or **thick** according to the amount of dermis included (Fig. 3.2).

These various categories of graft are not really completely distinct one from the other. They merely represent convenient reference points on a continuous scale of decreasing thickness from the whole skin graft to the graft consisting of little more than epidermis. The real difference in practice is between the whole skin graft and the split-skin graft. The whole skin graft is cut with a scalpel while the split-skin graft, of whatever thickness, is usually cut with a special instrument.

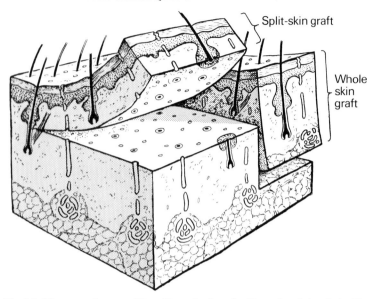

Fig. 3.1 The two main types of free skin graft, the split-skin graft and the whole skin graft, showing the constituents of each.

The whole skin graft, once cut, leaves behind no epidermal structure in the donor area from which resurfacing can take place; the split-skin graft leaves adnexal remnants, pilo-sebaceous follicle or sweat gland apparatus, as foci from which the donor site can resurface. As a result the donor area of a split-skin graft heals spontaneously and requires no care other than that usually accorded any raw surface; the donor area of a whole skin graft has to be closed by direct suture or, if it is too large for this, covered with a split-skin graft. This limits the size of the whole skin graft which can usefully be cut in practice. Extensive defects are split-skin grafted; the whole skin graft is restricted to small defects.

While the properties of the whole skin graft are relatively constant, those of the split-skin graft depend in some degree on the thickness of its dermal component, the thicker split-skin graft approximating to the whole skin graft in its characteristics.

The whole skin graft takes less readily than the split-skin graft and before it can be used successfully conditions must be optimal. The thinner the split-skin graft the better are its chances of taking in difficult conditions.

The stability of a graft depends on dermis and so the thicker graft stands late trauma better than the thin graft.

The whole skin graft remains virtually at its original size; the

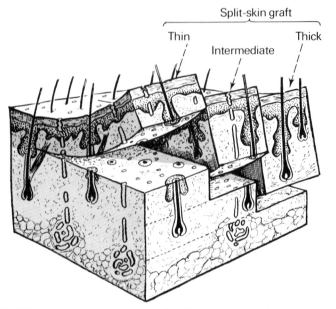

Fig. 3.2 The varying thicknesses of the split-skin graft, showing the constituents of each.

split-skin graft tends to contract if circumstances permit, e.g. inside the mouth or across a flexure. Within broad limits the thinner a graft the more it will contract secondarily.

During its transfer from donor to recipient site a free skin graft is completely, even if only temporarily, detached from the body. While so detached such a graft remains viable for a limited period whose precise limit depends on the ambient temperature (see p. 98). To survive permanently it has to become reattached and obtain a fresh blood supply from its new habitat. The various processes which result in its reattachment and revascularisation are collectively called **take**.

THE PROCESS OF TAKE

The graft initially adheres to its new bed by fibrin and its immediate nutritional requirements appear to be met by diffusion from the plasma which exudes from the bed providing a so-called **plasmatic circulation**. This is rapidly reinforced by the outgrowth of capillary buds from the recipient area to unite with those on the deep surface of the graft (Fig. 3.3). This link-up is usually well advanced by the third day. It is said to be reinforced by fresh ingrowing vessels from

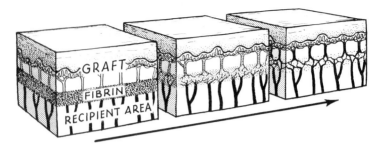

Fig. 3.3 A diagrammatic representation of graft take, showing the initial anchorage by fibrin, the commencing organisation of the fibrin clot with ingrowth of capillaries from graft bed and graft and the linking-up of the vessels with conversion of the fibrin into a fibrous tissue attachment.

the graft bed so that the vascular pattern of the graft is re-organised but the evidence for this is not very substantial.

Coincidentally with the vascular link-up the fibrin is infiltrated by fibroblasts which gradually convert the initial, rather tenuous, adhesion of the fibrin clot into a more effective definitive attachment by fibrous tissue. The strength of this attachment increases quickly, providing within four days an anchorage which allows the graft to be handled safely if reasonable care is taken. More slowly a lymphatic link-up is added and even more slowly nerve supply is re-established, though imperfectly and not invariably.

Of these various processes the ones most relevant in clinical practice are the provision of the blood supply and the fibrous tissue fixation. The speed and effectiveness with which they are provided are determined by the characteristics of the **bed** on which the graft is laid, the characteristics of the **graft** itself and the **conditions under which the graft is applied to the bed**.

The graft bed
The bed must have a rich enough blood supply to vascularise the graft as rapidly as possible and also be capable of providing the necessary fibrin anchorage.

Vascularisation
This is achieved by the outgrowth of capillary buds and the more rapid the process and profuse the outgrowth the more suitable the particular surface is for grafting. Capillary outgrowth is also the key factor in the production of granulation tissue and here, too, speed and profusion of outgrowth determines the effectiveness of the process. With capillary outgrowth common to both processes the

surgeon can assess the suitability of a surface for grafting by considering the speed with which it would be expected to granulate, left ungrafted. *The potential recipient area incapable of producing granulations will not take a free skin graft* (Fig. 3.4). *The surface which granulates rapidly and well takes a graft readily; one which granulates poorly takes a graft less readily.*

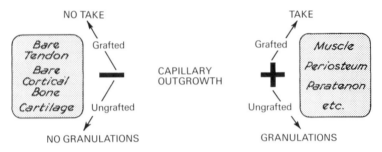

Fig. 3.4 Capillary outgrowth as the common factor in the development of granulations on various surfaces and their capacity to take free skin grafts.

Soft tissues, such as muscle and fascia, in general accept grafts readily but the ease with which fat can be grafted varies with the site. On the face, fat is extremely vascular and grafts easily; elsewhere its relatively poor vascularity makes it a poorer surface to graft. Cartilage covered with perichondrium, bone covered with periosteum and tendon covered with paratenon, whether parietal or visceral, all accept grafts readily.

Bare cartilage and bare tendon cannot be relied on to take a graft (Fig. 3.5) though if the area is small, the blood supply of the surrounding tissue may be sufficiently profuse to allow the graft in its vascularisation to bridge the defect and cover it successfully (p. 62).

Bone requires more detailed consideration because its behaviour varies in different sites. Bare cortical bone as typified by outer table of skull (Fig. 3.5) or subcutaneous border of tibia lacks sufficient vascularity to take a graft successfully. The hard palate and the bony orbit are both capable of taking grafts. The bone of the diploë, exposed when the outer table of the skull has been removed, and medullary bone generally, will also take a graft successfully. In each instance the ease of graft take parallels the speed and effectiveness with which each would granulate left denuded.

Fibrin anchorage

Any surface suitable for grafting on the basis of its vascular

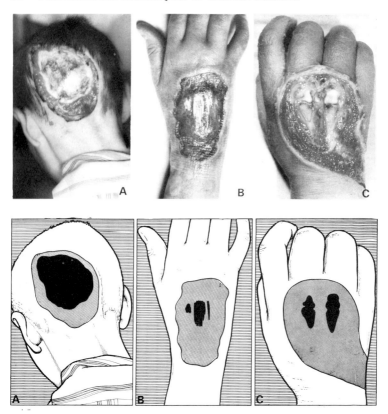

Fig. 3.5 Typical areas—*shown in black*—which will not take a graft successfully.

A   Bare cortical outer table of skull.
B   Bare tendon of extensor digitorum.
C   Bare cortex of metacarpals and proximal phalanges with articular cartilage and open metacarpophalangeal joints.

characteristics has fibrinogen and the enzymes which convert it into fibrin in adequate quantities to provide the necessary adhesion unless the surface is harbouring organisms which destroy fibrin. The organism *par excellence* which does this is the *Str. pyogenes*, probably by virtue of its potent fibrinolysin. This problem arises mainly when granulating surfaces are being grafted. It is discussed on p. 84.

The graft
Skin grafts can vary both in their thickness and the vascularity of the skin from which they are taken. Each of these variables affects their speed of vascularisation and consequently the ease with which they take.

Variations in graft thickness relate to the thickness of their dermal component and this influences their vascularity, dermis in general being less vascular in its deeper part. The number of cut capillary ends exposed when a thick skin graft is cut is smaller than with a thin graft (Fig. 3.18) and the full thickness graft has even fewer. With vascularisation slower the thicker the graft, thin grafts are generally easier to get to take than thick grafts. In order to get the thickest grafts to take, conditions have to be little short of ideal. These facts apply to grafts taken from sites other than the head and neck—the abdomen, thigh, arm, buttock, etc. The head and neck sites commonly used as donor areas have such a rich blood supply that full thickness grafts from one of these sites compare very favourably in their vascular characteristics with thin split-skin grafts taken from elsewhere.

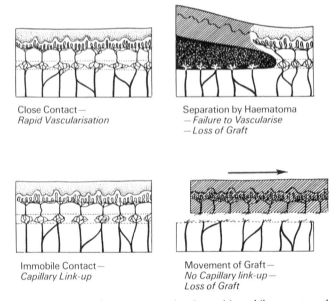

Close Contact—
Rapid Vascularisation

Separation by Haematoma
—Failure to Vascularise
—Loss of Graft

Immobile Contact—
Capillary Link-up

Movement of Graft—
No Capillary link-up—
Loss of Graft

Fig. 3.6 The influence of accurate approximation and immobile contact on the vascularisation of a graft.

Conditions for take

Rapid vasciularisation is all-important and the distance to be travelled by the capillary buds in order to link-up clearly needs to be as short as possible; the graft has therefore to be in the closest possible contact with the bed. The most frequent cause of separation is bleeding from the bed, the consequent haematoma acting as a block to link-up of the outgrowing capillaries (Fig. 3.6).

At the same time the graft has to lie immobile on the bed until it is firmly attached. In particular, shearing strains which tend to make the graft slide to and fro are to be avoided (Fig. 3.6) until the initial fibrin adhesion has been converted into a strong fibrous tissue anchorage.

In summary, *given a bed capable of providing the necessary capillary outgrowth to vascularise a graft and free of graft destroying pathogens inimical to graft take, the conditions necessary for successful take are close, immobile contact between graft and bed.* Grafts are usually lost because of haematoma which separates the graft from its bed and/or shearing movements which prevent adhesion between graft and bed, each in its own way preventing capillary link-up and hence vascularisation. The methods used in clinical grafting practice vary according to the clinical situation but in each instance the particular method adopted is used because it is considered to be the one most likely to prevent haematoma and avoid shearing movement.

The phenomenon of bridging

A graft may survive over bare cortical bone, tendon or cartilage, and even if separated from its graft bed by blood clot, provided always that the area is small enough. In such circumstances the graft survives by bridging (Fig. 3.7), a phenomenon of particular interest in view of the light which it throws on the process of vascularisation. It provides confirmatory evidence of a link-up with the existing vascular network of the graft since bridging could not occur if vascularisation took place solely by capillary invasion from the graft bed.

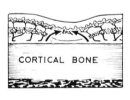
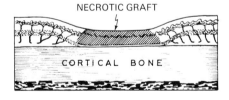

Successful bridging of small defect

Failure to bridge larger defect

Fig. 3.7 The phenomenon of bridging.

In most circumstances bridging is strictly limited in area and beyond this necrosis will occur. Certainly it cannot be relied on to cover bone, tendon or cartilage successfully. Where a very rich vascular network exists both in a graft and its bed, however, bridging may be possible over a much larger area and the composite free graft of ear skin and cartilage for alar defects succeeds or fails largely on the extent to which bridging is successful.

THE WHOLE SKIN GRAFT

The whole skin graft requires optimal conditions to take successfully and so cannot be applied for example to a granulating area. A graft of relatively small size only can be used for its donor site must either be closed by suture or covered with a split-skin graft. These adverse qualities naturally limit its usefulness in practice.

Its desirable properties on the other hand make it very much the graft of choice in certain circumstances. It does not contract secondarily and this makes it suitable for skin replacement around the mouth and eyelids, and on the palmar aspect of hand and fingers. It stands pressure well and so is useful on the sole of the foot. In the face moreover a whole skin graft from one of the more suitable donor sites described below will give in general the best colour and texture match.

DONOR SITES

The thickness, appearance, texture and vascularity of skin vary greatly in different parts of the body and have a strong influence on the selection of the donor site appropriate to a particular surgical situation.

Postauricular skin
The posterior surface of the ear and the adjoining postauricular hairless mastoid skin (Fig. 3.8) make the best donor site when the face is being grafted. The one disadvantage is the limited quantity of skin available and this restricts its use very materially. It gives a most excellent skin colour and texture match (Fig. 3.9) and when replacing eyelid skin is often virtually undetectable. The vascularity both of the graft and the sites to which it is usually applied make it the easiest of whole skin grafts to get to take. The donor site is closed by direct suture.

The postauricular whole skin graft has its main use in repairing small defects of the face and the area of skin available behind the ear alone limits the size of the defect which it can be used to cover.

Upper eyelid
In the adult a small area of skin is nearly always available on the

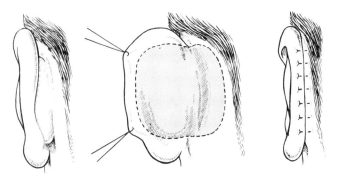

Fig. 3.8 The area within which postauricular skin is available and the method of closing the resultant defect.

upper eyelid and this can be useful particularly for another eyelid. The colour and texture match is naturally outstandingly good but the area available is extremely limited unless there is marked redundancy of the upper eyelid skin.

Supraclavicular skin
The skin of the lower posterior triangle of the neck (Fig. 3.10) gives a good colour and texture match used on the face though one distinctly inferior to postauricular skin. A large area of skin is available but the increase is too small to make it more obviously useful as the donor area itself must be grafted in many instances. This adds a cosmetic effect of its own and one which is likely to be particularly undesirable in the female where the donor area is so often exposed.

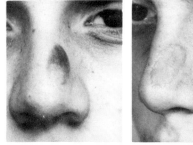
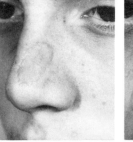
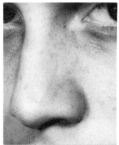

Fig. 3.9 The early and late appearance of a postauricular full thickness graft applied to the nose following the excision of a simple pigmented naevus.

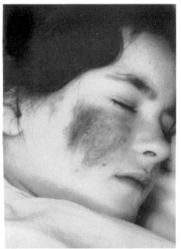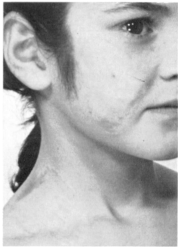

Fig. 3.10 The late appearance of a supraclavicular full thickness graft applied to the face following excision of a hairy naevus. The supraclavicular defect was covered with a dermatome split-skin graft from abdomen.

Its usefulness is thus rather restricted and it is not often needed. It might be considered for a defect just too large for a postauricular whole skin graft where a rotation flap is contra-indicated.

Flexural skin
The antecubital fossa and the groin are both described as possible donor sites. The dermis is thin and the skin mobile on the deeper tissues. Applied to the face the cosmetic result is not greatly inferior to that using supraclavicular skin. Only a limited quantity is available unless a secondary graft is used to cover the donor site.

In the antecubital fossa the donor site is more often exposed and the scarring of closure consequently more of a drawback. Furthermore, if much tension is used in closing it by direct suture a hypertrophic scar or keloid may develop. Its use as a donor site is not recommended. In the groin the pubic hair may limit both the use and quantity available but the area is valuable if a long narrow graft is needed, for closure in such circumstances is relatively simple. For the hand it provides a good source of skin.

Thigh and abdominal skin
The texture and colour match of thigh and abdominal skin grafted to the face is usually poor. The skin either stays extremely pale or

becomes hyperpigmented relative to the rest of the face. An added defect is a loss of the constantly varying fine play of normal facial expression. The grafted area has instead a rather mask-like appearance due possibly to its thicker dermis. Although a thick split-skin graft cut from the abdomen with the drum dermatome tends to be used rather than a whole skin graft for replacing extensive areas of facial skin loss it shares the defects of the whole skin graft.

Both sites provide a good source of skin for the palm of the hand and the thick dermis gives a good pad to take the necessary pressure used on the sole of the foot. If a graft of any size is used the donor site must in its turn be grafted and even when the donor site can be directly sutured the scar usually stretches badly.

METHOD OF USE

The whole skin graft is accurately fitted to the defect and so a pattern of the defect to be grafted must be made to have the graft at normal skin tension in its new site. Aluminium foil, jaconet, and polythene sheet are all useful materials for making patterns. Around the eyelids aluminium foil is probably best; elsewhere the others are more satisfactory (Fig. 3.11).

The pattern of the area to be grafted is made before excision or after whichever is more convenient. If the defect is irregular, matching points can be tattooed with Bonney's Blue on the defect and on the graft before it is cut. When the pattern can only be made once the defect is surgically created, the defect should be displayed to the full before making the pattern. This applies with particular force to the eyelid where failure to make the pattern and subsequently the graft of a size to fill the defect in full will result in residual ectropion.

CUTTING THE GRAFT

In cutting a whole skin graft (Fig. 3.12) time and care can be spent at the actual time of cutting so that no fat is left on the graft, or the graft may be cut without special regard to fat, the fat being subsequently removed with scissors. Excision of the fat after the graft has been cut is a tedious business but to cut the graft without fat requires both skill and care. It is probably easier for the surgeon who seldom uses the method not to attempt it lest the graft be buttonholed in the process. Most surgeons gradually acquire a feel for the correct plane at the time of cutting the graft.

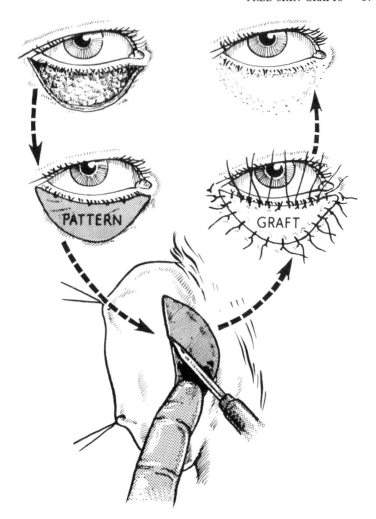

Fig. 3.11 The use of a pattern in cutting a whole skin graft to accurately fit the defect.

A useful device, especially in the concavity behind the ear, is to balloon the whole area with fluid, usually 1 in 200,000 noradrenaline. Using the pattern already made the outline is marked on the skin with Bonney's Blue, incised and undercut. It often helps to pull the skin of the graft taut over the knife with hooks so that the knife is cutting blindly, largely by touch. Alternatively, the graft can be held turned back so that cutting is done under vision. Oddly enough this method is less precise and usually results in more fat being left on

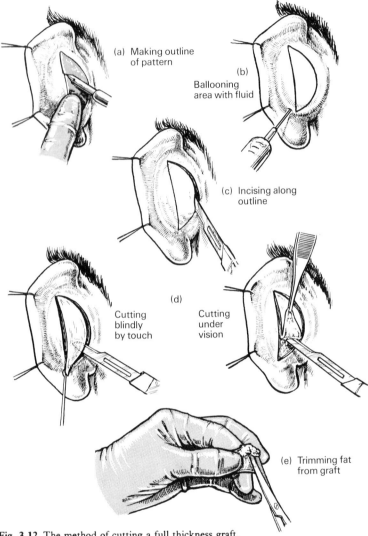

(a) Making outline of pattern

(b) Ballooning area with fluid

(c) Incising along outline

(d) Cutting blindly by touch   Cutting under vision

(e) Trimming fat from graft

Fig. 3.12 The method of cutting a full thickness graft.

the graft. Any fat left on the graft must be carefully removed with scissors.

CARE OF THE DONOR SITE

Behind the ear, closure by direct suture is usually feasible. Elsewhere direct suture should be used where possible. In the thigh and abdomen, where the superficial fascia is relatively fixed, the exposed fascia is best excised to facilitate closure. In the flexures, where the skin is much more mobile, this is less often necessary. Where the donor site defect is too large to suture a split-skin graft must be used to cover it.

THE SPLIT-SKIN GRAFT

A split-skin graft may vary in thickness from what is virtually a whole skin graft to one which is almost epidermal and each has its place depending on which property of the particular thickness is wanted. It is used either as temporary cover to provide healing, e.g. in burns, in the immediate postexcision treatment of skin malignancies, in the coverage of bridge pedicle defects, or as permanent cover. In general temporary grafts are cut thinner than permanent grafts but not infrequently a graft meant for temporary cover proves entirely acceptable as permanent cover.

DONOR SITES

These are selected in any set instance by such factors as the amount of skin required; whether a good colour and texture match is needed; local convenience, as in grafting from forearm to hand with need for only one dressing; the necessity of having no hair on the graft; the cutting instrument available; the desirability where possible of avoiding the leg in the aged or outpatient.

The usual areas are:

1. Virtually the whole of the reasonably plane surface of the torso.
2. The thigh and upper arm.
3. The flexor aspect of forearm.

When these are not available or all possible sites are needed skin can also be cut from:

1. The other aspects of forearm.
2. The lower leg.

GRAFT-CUTTING INSTRUMENTS

The instruments commonly used for cutting grafts are:

1. The Humby knife which was developed from and has now largely replaced the Blair knife.
2. The drum dermatome.
3. The electric dermatome.

The Humby and Blair knives (Fig. 3.13)
The first split-skin grafts were taken with the Blair knife. It had a long, straight-edged blade and was something of a virtuoso instrument, grafts of a consistently correct thickness being extremely difficult to cut. With the advent of the Humby knife, a version having the added refinement of an adjustable roller to control the thickness of the graft cut, the Blair knife is seldom used. Like the Blair knife, the Humby knife can only be used on convex surfaces but despite this it is the most frequently used instrument for routine graft cutting. Of the versions now on the market, the Watson modification is the best.

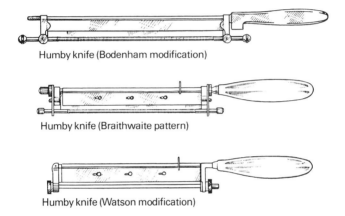

Humby knife (Bodenham modification)

Humby knife (Braithwaite pattern)

Humby knife (Watson modification)

Fig. 3.13 The modified Humby knives.

Placing the donor site
The donor site most often used is the thigh and the positioning of the leg for this purpose will be described in detail (Fig. 3.14) but the principles outlined can be applied to any other donor site.

The leg is placed with the appropriate group of muscles relaxed so that by pressing the muscle group either medially or laterally the maximum of plane surface is presented to the knife.

For the **medial side of thigh** the leg is placed as in Figure 3.14. The assistant presses from below with the flat of both hands pushing round the hamstrings and adductors to give the necessary wide flat surface for cutting a broad graft.

When the **lateral aspect** is used (Fig. 3.14) the surface produced when the assistant presses laterally is less satisfactorily flat than the medial aspect especially in its lower part because of the tautness of the iliotibial band. The depression which it produces between the

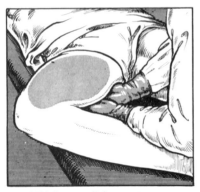

Thigh—*medial aspect*

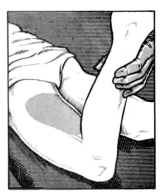

Thigh—*posterior aspect*
(patient prone)

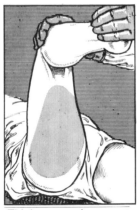

Thigh—*posterior aspect*
(patient lying on back)

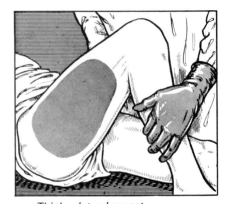

Thigh—*lateral aspect*

Fig. 3.14 Positioning the thigh for cutting a graft.

vastus lateralis and the biceps femoris becomes less noticeable proximally.

For the **posterior aspect** (Fig. 3.14) flexion of both hip and knee are needed to get at the surface unless the subject is prone. Distally the ridges produced by the diverging hamstrings make a good graft difficult to obtain but passing proximally the flat surface broadens and a good graft can be cut readily.

Because of the prominence of the femoral shaft the **anterior aspect** does not give a broad plane surface and it is not used unless all donor sites are needed or a narrow graft is specifically desired.

In the **arm** (Fig. 3.15), positioning and pressure are used in the same way to give the broadest plane surface.

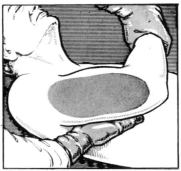

Upper Arm—*lateral aspect*

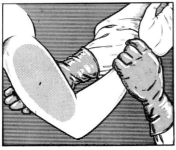

Upper Arm—*medial aspect*

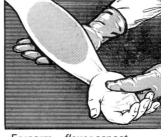

Forearm—*flexor aspect*

Fig. 3.15 Positioning the arm for cutting a graft.

Preparing the knife

Ideally the blade when cutting moves to and fro smoothly over the skin surface which does not move at all with the knife. Drag, which is the result of friction between blade and skin, causes the skin to oscillate to and fro with the knife and makes the graft more difficult to cut. It cannot be completely eliminated but lubrication does help to reduce it. An excellent lubricant is liquid paraffin and the surface of the blade next the skin should be smeared with it. When the Humby knife is used the lubricant must be kept clear of the roller lest the graft instead of gathering on the blade as it passes between blade and roller should stick to the roller, winding itself around it.

Setting the knife

Setting the knife is necessary only with the Humby knife where graft thickness is controlled by adjusting the distance between roller and blade. The advantage of the interchangeable blade which is now almost universal is that it gives a much cleaner cut with minimal drag from bluntness, but this is to some extent offset by the slight lack of rigidity of the blade which is thin and only partly supported. As a result the adjustment markings present on the knife give a setting which tends to vary with different blades and reliance on the markings alone in setting the roller will give inconsistence of graft thickness.

By holding the knife up to the light the actual clearance between blade and roller can be seen and this method gives a more reliable reading. Although the surgeon learns with experience to set the knife by eye a clearance of a little less than $\frac{1}{2}$ mm as a rule will be found to give a graft of average thickness. It must be emphasised however that this must in turn be controlled by watching both the graft as it is cut and the bed from which it is being cut. The guiding characters of thickness are described below.

Cutting the graft

The surgeon should work from the more convenient side of the patient cutting down the limb or up according to his position.

A little in front of the knife and moving smoothly at a fixed distance from it a wooden board is held pressed down on the skin (Fig. 3.16). The board serves the double purpose of steadying and flattening the skin as the blade reaches it. The edge of the board

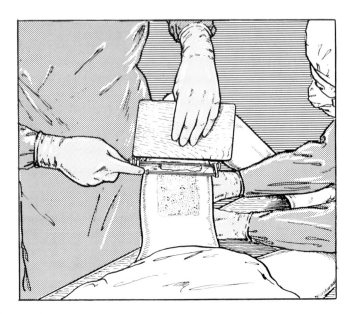

Fig. 3.16 Cutting a graft with the Humby knife.

which is pressing on the skin is lubricated with liquid paraffin so that it moves smoothly with the knife. To get knife and board moving smoothly forward in unison takes practice.

With both Blair and Humby knife the secret of good cutting is to concentrate on an even to and fro motion rather than on the forward moving of the knife as it cuts the graft.

It may help to make the whole skin area as taut as possible by having a further assistant hold the skin steady and tight with a wooden board just behind the knife before it starts to cut. The board is kept still as the knife moves forward to cut the graft. Where the skin is atrophic, lax and mobile as in the aged or emaciated subject this manoeuvre is useful insofar as it helps to eliminate drag.

With the Bodenham modification the clearance between roller and blade is apt to increase as the graft is being cut so that it becomes steadily thicker and this must be watched for so that the roller can be readjusted to its original setting. The Braithwaite pattern is less prone to this and the roller mechanism of the recently introduced Watson modification is virtually free of this defect.

Assessment of thickness

Although a setting of the roller has been suggested above, the surgeon must be prepared to modify it if necessary. The first 6 mm or so of the graft cut gives a good indication of the thickness and the setting can be adjusted accordingly.

The **translucency of the graft** is the main index of thickness (Fig. 3.17). The very thin graft is translucent and not unlike tissue paper; the grey of the knife blade shows easily through. Thicker grafts are increasingly opaque until the whole skin graft has the colour and appearance of cadaver skin. A split-skin graft of intermediate thickness is moderately translucent.

The **pattern of bleeding of the donor site** gives a further indication of thickness (Fig. 3.18). The thin graft produces a high density of tiny bleeding points; the thicker graft gives a lower density of larger points.

While these criteria are generally applicable they should always be correlated with the initial appearance of the skin in the individual patient particularly as to the presence of clinical atrophy. With the papery skin of the aged the graft must be correspondingly thin and the distribution of bleeding points gives no help in such cases.

The thickness of the skin also seems to vary in different parts of the limb; in general lateral is thicker than medial and distal thicker than proximal, but individual variation is considerable.

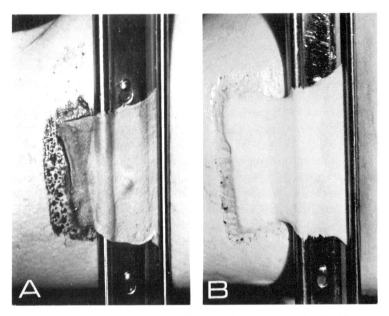

Fig. 3.17 The translucency of a thin split-skin graft (A), and a thick split-skin graft (B).

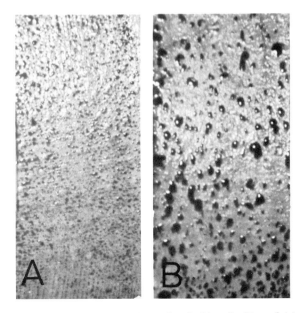

Fig. 3.18 The pattern of bleeding of the donor site of a thin split-skin graft (A), and a thick split-skin graft (B).

The drum dermatome

In Great Britain the model generally used is the Padgett-Hood or one of its modifications (Fig. 3.19). Its clumsiness and uncertainty in use compared with the Humby knife has prevented it from achieving great popularity for routine purposes. An added defect is that successive drums of skin are not readily cut without meticulous cleansing and fresh preparation of both dermatome and skin. None of these criticisms apply to the Reese dermatome which is currently popular in the United States and which is a much superior instrument. It is unfortunately not manufactured in this country. The description which follows refers only to the Padgett-Hood instrument or its modifications and not the Reese dermatone.

Although the drum dermatome is not used routinely there are occasions where its use is particularly indicated. The precise indications naturally depend to some extent on the relative skill of the

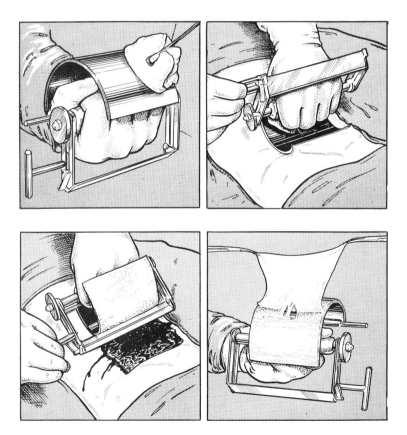

Fig. 3.19 Cutting a graft with the drum dermatome.

operator with dermatome and grafting knife but in most cases the Humby knife is preferred unless there is a positive reason for using the dermatome. In the extensive deep burn where all donor areas are needed the dermatome may have to be used since at least until the advent of the electric dermatome it alone could cut from abdomen, chest and much of back. On the credit side, the dermatome graft is recognisably uniform in thickness and this gives it a cosmetic advantage over skin cut with the Humby knife when the face is being grafted. It is in providing extensive skin cover for the face that the dermatome graft finds its main use and in those circumstances a thick split-skin graft is used.

In using the dermatome the drum and donor area are painted with an adhesive compound. Where the drum is pressed against the skin the two surfaces adhere and the skin can be lifted with the drum for cutting by the knife blade which is moved to and fro parallel to the axis of the drum at a previously adjusted, fixed clearance distance. As cutting proceeds the graft is left adhering to the drum (Fig. 3.19).

Cutting a graft with the dermatome can only be learned by demonstration and practice and it is not proposed to discuss the technique in any detail. There are some hints, however, which may help the beginner.

Graft thickness

Most instruments have a gauge which determines thickness. A graft of medium thickness is 12 to 14/1000 inch, but thickness from 8 or even less up to 16 or 18 can be used according to need. As with the Humby knife the gauge reading is not always accurate and it should always be matched against the graft actually cut. It is often difficult to see the graft well early on in the cut but almost as good an indication is the density and size of the bleeding points of the donor area. A thick graft is technically easier to cut than a thin one. When lobules of fat appear the graft is in effect of whole skin graft thickness.

Lacquering the surfaces

Both drum and skin should be given a thorough preliminary cleansing with ether to remove all grease so that the lacquer will stick properly. Smooth application of the lacquer helps it to dry uniformly. The edges of the drum take the greatest pull when the dermatome is cutting and should be carefully lacquered. Being colder than the skin as a rule the drum dries more slowly but patience in waiting until the surfaces are quite dry pays dividends.

Lubrication

Both the surface of the knife moving against the skin and the axle of the drum should be smeared with liquid paraffin to help the knife to move smoothly to and fro. Lubricant must not get on to either of the lacquered surfaces or complete loss of stickiness will result.

Cutting the graft

A good initial cut of the knife blade usually means a good graft and care with the first cut is worth while, making sure especially that the skin is sticking from side to side of the drum. Just how far the drum can safely be raised to pull up the skin for cutting depends on the laxity of the skin. Raising the drum too little allows the knife to plough deeply into the skin beyond the side of the drum and an assistant should be ready to depress the skin here with a suitable instrument. Raising the drum too far increases the tension unduly and is liable to tear the skin from the drum so that the knife cannot cut properly and this produces a patchy, incomplete drum of skin. The middle course is only acquired with experience as is the co-ordinated to and fro cutting of the knife and forward rolling of the drum.

Removing the skin from the drum

The lacquer remains largely on the graft and as it is taken from the drum its stickiness must be removed. With mosquito forceps on each corner to elevate the margin of the graft an ether swab will remove the lacquer as the graft comes off the drum. This method is effective but messy and a cleaner way is to spray the graft coming off the drum with either penicillin or sulpha powder. The lacquer remains on the graft but has lost its stickiness.

The problem of residual lacquer on the graft has largely been solved recently by using Evo-Stik 'Impact' household adhesive. This contact adhesive can readily be diluted to a viscosity suitable for application to drum and skin by adding an equal volume of ether and stirring until the two liquids are well mixed. As an adhesive it is much better than any the author has previously used and it has the added advantage of bonding to the drum even more strongly than to the skin so that the graft strips off the drum completely clean leaving the adhesive entirely on the drum.

The electric dermatome

One of the major disadvantages of the electric dermatome is that it is at once a complex and fragile instrument. It does not stand rough handling and if anything goes wrong it has to go back to the maker with all the annoyance and delay which this entails. With it much of the skill has gone from graft cutting and if the instructions are carefully followed the surgeon can scarcely fail to cut a graft successfully. It has the great merit too of cutting a graft of controlled width and accurately controllable thickness from almost any part of trunk or limbs and readily cuts a very thin graft—a thing that other instruments do less successfully.

In appearance it is not unlike a large hair-cutting machine (Fig. 3.20) and the resemblance is maintained in action with the rapidly oscillating cutting blade which is driven either electrically or by compressed air. The skin is held steady and lubricated with liquid paraffin so that the instrument can move forward smoothly.

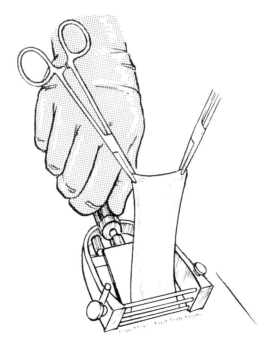

Fig. 3.20 Cutting a graft with the electric dermatome.

It is in the grafting of the extensive deep burn that the electric dermatome has been a very real advance. Its ability to cut skin from almost any part of the body surface has greatly extended the available donor areas. The straight margin and uniform thickness of the graft which it cuts mean that a limb can be flayed with scarcely any wastage of skin between adjoining graft sites in the knowledge that the whole donor area will heal uniformly and rapidly. It becomes a practical possibility as a result to cut successive crops of skin from the same donor site, a most valuable property when skin is at a premium.

HEALING OF THE DONOR AREA (Fig. 3.21)

In the donor site of a split-skin graft greater or lesser portions of the pilosebaceous apparatus and sweat glands remain, and from these multiple foci epithelium spreads until the area is covered with skin. The pilosebaceous apparatus is much more active as a centre of epithelial regeneration than the sweat gland which reacts more sluggishly. Anatomically the sweat glands extend more deeply than the hair follicles and this is reflected in the different healing patterns of sites from which thin and thick split-skin grafts have been cut. The donor site of the thin graft on the one hand with its full complement of cut hair follicles heals rapidly within 7 to 9 days, while the donor site of the thick graft on the other hand, depending entirely on sweat gland remnants, heals much more slowly, taking 14 days or more. Most grafts are of intermediate thickness and leave a percentage of follicles so that healing takes 10 to 14 days. A donor area only granulates if no follicles or sweat glands remain and in such

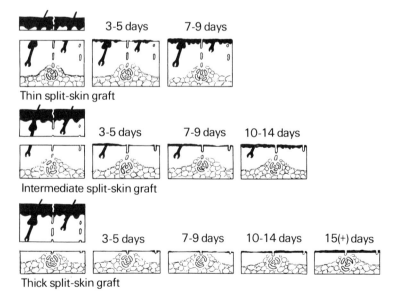

Fig. 3.21 The healing of the donor sites of the various thicknesses of split-skin graft.

circumstances healing must take place from the margin of the area.

It will be seen from this that the healing of a donor area is analogous to that of a superficial burn.

CARE OF THE DONOR AREA

The main difficulty in treating a donor site arises from the fact that the dressing becomes extremely hard and sticks like glue to the skin so that its removal causes bleeding and considerable pain as the regenerating epithelium is torn off. Usual practice is to leave the dressing quite alone until it separates spontaneously or, failing this, to soak it off. Such masterly inactivity is only possible if the dressing remains dry. When part of the graft has been thicker the corresponding segment of donor area heals less rapidly and may even granulate with resulting discharge. It has then to be treated as a granulating wound. If small in area it will heal spontaneously, but if of any size it should be grafted without delay.

A useful prophylactic where all or part of a donor area looks at all doubtful from the depth point of view and particularly if fat is showing to any extent is to cover it with a thin split-skin graft when the initial graft is cut.

Various semi-occlusive dressings have recently been introduced for use on donor areas as a result of the experimental finding that the donor area which is not permitted to dry heals faster. To date they have not been uniformly successful in clinical use.

A late problem which can arise in relation to donor areas is the development of hypertrophic scarring. This most often affects the abdomen, inner aspect of thigh and buttock, though any donor site can be affected. One's impression, difficult to prove, is that the thicker the graft cut and the younger the patient the greater its proneness to occur. Warning of its imminent development is a complaint of severe itching of the donor area. Itching, although it can occur independently, is more often a precursor of hypertrophic change.

Left untreated, the condition does eventually settle down but at the expense of a white, ugly atrophic-looking patch of scarred skin. A definite clinical impression, again difficult to prove, is that the use of one of the locally active steroids in ointment form reduces both the incidence of the complication and its severity. It certainly relieves the itch consistently and is probably best applied as soon as itch is complained of and continued until the area is showing signs of settling, as indicated by its clinical appearance.

THE RECIPIENT AREA

Free skin grafts are applied either to raw surfaces surgically created or at least surgically clean, or to granulating wounds. The practice of grafting varies with the two types of surface as does preparation for grafting.

THE SURGICALLY CLEAN SURFACE

Preparing the recipient area

Although a whole skin graft or split-skin graft may be used according to circumstance the underlying principle does not vary. A level surface is always desirable for irregularities are likely to give rise to tenting of the graft across the hollow unless it is shallow. The common reason for failure of a graft where it might reasonably be expected to take well is **haematoma** and a completely dry field is essential before the graft is applied. To achieve this several measures are used.

Infiltration of the area prior to excision. Bleeding can be reduced by injecting a vasoconstricting fluid into the tissue to be excised. The fluid usually used is local anaesthetic with adrenaline but as some of the local anaesthetics are vasodilators it is preferable in the generally anaesthetised patient to use saline as the diluent. Either adrenaline or noradrenaline can be used. Noradrenaline is a weaker constrictor of cutaneous vessels than adrenaline but it is less likely to have central effects after absorption. Considerable variation in recommended concentrations are described but in the large volumes often required in plastic surgery concentrations of 1 part in 200,000 of saline are safe and in practice effective.

Ligature of obvious bleeding points. The forceps must pick up only the actual point so that the necrosis caused by the short fine catgut tie is minimal. Diathermy is a possible alternative and in practice take is not significantly reduced if the block of tissue killed by either method is small enough.

Local adrenaline. If the tissue excised has not already been infiltrated local adrenaline or noradrenaline will reduce capillary ooze.

Use of time. Without doubt time is the most important single factor in haemostasis. The steps of the operation should be planned to give the recipient area the longest possible time for the normal haemostatic processes to become effective. While waiting for bleeding to cease the area may be left covered with gauze soaked in saline or adrenaline, or alternatively it may be irrigated with adrenaline solution and then left exposed. What must be avoided is constant dabbing and swabbing which only serve to encourage oozing.

Use and misuse of the sucker. The sucker can play a most valuable part during excision for it allows the surgeon to see precisely where he is cutting. The defect once created however, suction applied to the raw area only keeps bleeding going. If a specific clot has to be sucked off, the sucker nozzle should never actually touch the tissue or the bleeding point will surely begin again.

When the graft had been sutured in position and the dressing is ready some surgeons suck out any clots which have formed during suturing. While this is not ineffective, the dressing must be applied without delay for bleeding usually begins again as a result of the trauma of the suction.

Marginal bleeders. For these a ligature is seldom needed. With appropriate placing the graft suture can be made to serve the double purpose of haemostasis and graft anchorage.

Irrigation and orange stick. Unless the graft bed is absolutely dry it is wise to flush out the whole site with saline once the graft is sutured in place using a 20 ml syringe with blunt cannula. Any small remaining clot can be removed by inserting an orange stick tipped with cotton wool. When the stick is twirled the clot is caught by the wool and can be removed with the stick.

THE GRANULATING AREA

In assessing a granulating area for grafting two factors are of importance—clinical appearance and bacterial flora.

Clinical appearance

Healthy granulations are flat, red and vascular, do not bleed unduly readily, and are free from a surface film of sloughing collagen. Good marginal healing is presumptive evidence that granulations will accept a graft for it can be assumed that infection virulent enough to destroy a graft would be inimical to marginal epithelial growth.

Unsatisfactory granulations take several forms:

1. Granulations left ungrafted for any length of time become more fibrous and less vascular so that it becomes increasingly difficult to get a graft to take. Infection tends to add to the difficulties of grafting in those circumstances.

2. When subjected to inadequate pressure, granulations tend to become oedematous and in this state are often miscalled exuberant. Such granulations need pressure rather than excision and copper

sulphate has certainly no place in the care of any surface which it is proposed to graft. Its only effect is to produce a coagulum which must be cast before a graft will take.

3. Haemorrhages are prone to take place into oedematous granulations producing a very typical clinical appearance.

4. The typically gelatinous haemorrhagic granulations harbouring *Streptococcus pyogenes*, which will be discussed later.

5. When a slough separates naturally the granulations left often have a tenacious film of necrotic collagen which is slow to separate and difficult to rub off.

Bacterial flora
Any of the common organisms may infect an area according to site and circumstance. With the exception of *Streptococcus pyogenes* and *Pseudomonas pyocyanea* such organisms are of little consequence as a general rule and clinical appearance is a better guide than bacterial flora in assessing suitability for grafting.

Streptococcus pyogenes
The presence of this organism is an absolute contra-indication to any grafting procedure; its possible presence necessitates routine bacteriological examination of exudate before grafting is contemplated. Why a graft should fail when it is present is not exactly known though interference with the normal fibrin attachment of the graft by the fibrinolysin which it produces may possibly be the cause.

Classically, granulations harbouring *Str. pyogenes* are glazed, gelatinous and bleed readily at the slightest touch; the marginal epithelium is seldom healthy and growing. With the routine use of antibiotics the classical picture may not be seen and the granulations may look quite healthy. But this deceptively tranquil behaviour of *Str. pyogenes* does not mitigate its destructive effect on grafts. It must always be eliminated before grafting is attempted.

Pseudomonas pyocyanea
Infection with this organism does reduce graft take but not to an extent comparable with *Str. pyogenes* and its presence is a nuisance rather than a disaster.

While *Ps. pyocyanea* infecting the surface of an extensive burn presents the problem of preventing systemic spread as well as that of controlling the local infection, systemic spread from less extensive raw surfaces is not a significant hazard and attention is more concerned with reducing or eliminating it as a step in preparing the granulations for grafting. Infection may be a mixed one with *Bacillus proteus* and in many instances the general measures for controlling local infection discussed under preparation of granulations for grafting are adequate. In any case while *Ps. pyocyanea* may reduce graft take by 5 to 10 per cent at most, grafting of the area does tend to end the infection. Grafting regardless of *Ps. pyocyanea* and accepting any small reduction in take gives excellent results.

In short a positive culture of *Ps. pyocyanea* is not a contra-indication to grafting if the granulations look otherwise healthy.

Other pathogens
The other pathogens which commonly infect wounds are *Staphylococcus aureus*, which in this situation is seldom more than a commensal, *Escherichia coli*, and *Bacillus proteus*. These latter two organisms are especially common in the badly handled, heavily contaminated, granulating wound. They are associated as a rule with a very typical, profuse, foul-smelling discharge and often occur as a mixed infection with *Ps. pyocyanea*. In the extensive deep burn they are often impossible to avoid but all too often they are allowed to contaminate quite small wounds from which they could be excluded by ordinary care.

Preparing granulations for grafting
It is axiomatic that the granulating area is being treated, not its flora, and so the role of local antibiotics is a controversial one. Antibiotics should not be used blindly on the basis of sensitivity reports. *Str. pyogenes* apart, the flora is immaterial provided the granulations look healthy and the fastest way to eliminate the flora is to graft the area.

In deciding the appropriate steps to eliminate *Str. pyogenes* from a granulating area the organism cannot be considered in isolation. Penicillin is the obvious antibiotic to use when it is the sole pathogen, for no resistant strains have been demonstrated. When it is associated with a penicillin resistant staphylococcus, the help of the bacteriologist should be invoked so that an antibiotic to which both are sensitive can be given, though in many situations an antiseptic such as chlorhexidine ('Hibitane') is simpler to use and more effective.

The main cause of continuing infection is the presence of slough; measures to get rid of it always reduce the infection. Surgical excision is the most rapid and effective method and in excising slough it pays to be as radical as is feasible. Excision to fascia is preferable to excision to fat. The alternative methods are natural separation unaided or helped by Eusol or the enzymatic agents for debridement.

Where a slough is separating naturally, pus is inevitable and is by no means undesirable for its autolytic enzymes play a valuable part in separating living from dead tissue. If there is no sign of invasive infection the flora is to be regarded as innocuous; only when the slough has gone is it possible to reduce the flora.

Enzymatic agents such as streptodornase-streptokinase and trypsin have been used but they have little to offer over the established methods. Eusol has still much to recommend it both for cleaning up dirty granulations and removing sloughs which are moist, diffluent, and difficult to exise cleanly. The Humby knife has been used with the roller widely open to excise both slough and heavily infected granulations and is most effective in the role, as is also the electric dermatome.

Granulations once clean and free of slough should be grafted without delay. During such waiting as is unavoidable an innocuous dressing which will not damage the granulations when removed should be used and tulle gras is usual. Unless *Str. pyogenes* is present an antibiotic is not essential. A meticulous dressings technique, adequate cover both in area and thickness of dressing, and infrequent dressings provide a better insurance against superadded infection than a blind reliance on antibiotics. The other factor which will keep granulations as healthy as possible for the longest time is pressure, and crepe bandages are usually necessary to provide this. Although the rationale is far from clear it is a common finding that hydrocortisone ointment sometimes improves unhealthy granulations or granulations showing little progress towards healing with or without grafts.

APPLICATION OF THE GRAFT

A skin graft can be applied in one of two ways. In the first method *pressure dressings* are applied to the graft; in the second the graft is left *exposed*. To appreciate the place of each method and make full use of the virtues peculiar to it, it is essential to see how each in its own way is fulfilling the conditions necessary for graft take. Only then can the correct method be selected as the one appropriate to a particular clinical situation.

To reiterate the conditions for successful graft take: *given a suitable bed, i.e. one capable of providing the capillary outgrowth to vascularise a graft and free of pathogens inimical to graft take* (see

p. 84), *the requirements for successful take are close and immobile contact between the graft and its bed.*

In practice grafts are lost because of *haematoma* separating the graft from its bed and *shearing movements* preventing adhesion between the graft and its bed. Each in its own way prevents capillary link-up. When the surgeon applies a graft in a particular clinical situation the method he adopts is consequently the one he feels is most likely to prevent haematoma and shearing movements.

It is proposed to discuss the principles which underlie the use of each method, pressure and exposed, and follow this by describing its actual practice. For convenience however the practice of grafting the granulating surface, whether using pressure methods or by exposure, will be discussed separately.

PRESSURE METHODS

When pressure is applied it is used as a means of providing the close attachment between the graft and its bed. The pressure is usually applied in one of two ways, usually both if the area is not a granulating surface. It is first applied directly and very precisely to the graft by means of a tie-over bolus dressing, the details of which will be described later. Suffice it to say at this stage that sutures are used. It is not used in granulating wounds because their edges do not hold sutures well.

Subsequent diffuse pressure dressings are applied which provide not merely added pressure but also, and possibly just as significantly, immobilisation making use of crepe bandaging or elastoplast. This type of pressure-immobilising dressing is relied on entirely when a granulating area is being grafted by the pressure method.

If further immobilisation is needed an added splint of plaster of Paris is used.

Applying the graft

The modes of application of a whole skin graft and a split-skin graft are similar in principle and in actual practice differ in only a few particulars. The sutures which fix the graft in position around its margin are left long and tied over a bolus of cotton wool which acts as a combined pressure and immobilising dressing. In this role it is reinforced by further dressings—gauze, cotton wool, and crepe bandages or elastoplast.

The whole skin graft

Cut to its prescribed pattern, the whole skin graft is intended to fit the defect accurately and so is carefully sutured edge to edge along its margin (Fig. 3.22). Enough sutures must be inserted to give as accurate an edge apposition as would be demanded in the suture of an incision and, just as in wound suture, care must be taken to avoid inversion of the edges. Only sufficient sutures are left long to provide a snug tie-over, the remainder are cut short.

The split-skin graft (Fig. 3.22)
The tendency of the split-skin graft to contract subsequently makes it advisable to display the raw area to the full so that as much skin

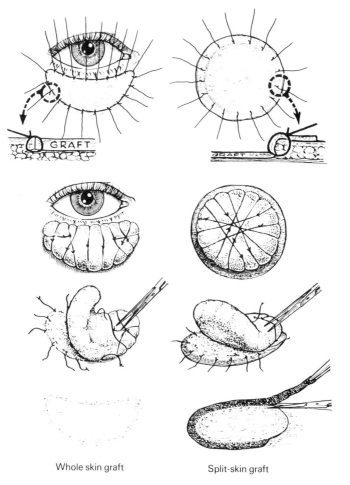

Whole skin graft   Split-skin graft

Fig. 3.22 The suturing and dressing of a whole skin graft and a split-skin graft showing the similarities and differences. Note the overlap of the split-skin graft being trimmed at the first dressing.

can be inserted as the defect is capable of taking. Such a graft is not usually spread on tulle gras before being applied to the raw area, though the added rigidity which the tulle gras backing provides does sometimes make handling of the graft technically easier.

The graft should be cut large enough to overlap the raw area slightly and there is no need to fit it accurately to the defect. It will take only to the margin of the defect in any case and the overlap can be trimmed off readily when the graft is dressed. If the margin is accurately sutured edge to edge it is apt to inroll and this gives a poor scar. The overlapping suture avoids this and also allows reduction of the number of sutures needed, for as long as the graft continues to overlap the defect between the sutures it will cover the raw area.

At one time this technique was used only when a good cosmetic result was not essential and in the face for example the graft was carefully sutured end to end. More recently, the overlapping method has been used even in the face with great simplification of technique and cosmetic results in no way inferior.

Dressing the graft (Fig. 3.22)

A layer of tulle gras laid over the graft before the tie-over cotton wool bolus is applied tends to ease the first postoperative dressing but is by no means essential. What is essential is the careful packing of the graft area with the cotton wool and this must be done meticulously so that the graft as a whole is subjected to uniform pressure. The bolus must be bulky and extend to the margin of the graft. The most efficient shape is probably one with a circular cross section which will spread the pressure evenly. With the wool tightly packed in position the long tie-over sutures are tied tightly over the dressing, anchoring dressing and graft in one mass.

The material best suited to act as a bolus is cotton wool prepared with flavine emulsion. Alternatives are cotton wool moistened with saline or tightly wrung out with liquid paraffin but flavine wool* is much to be preferred because of its fluffing properties.

Over further cotton wool padding to diffuse the pressure, crepe bandages are applied. If the site lends itself better to immobilisation

---

* PREPARATION OF FLAVINE WOOL. The materials used are flavine emulsion and best quality cotton wool or Gamgee. A sheet of cotton wool is soaked in the emulsion, previously warmed to reduce its viscosity, until it is completely impregnated. The excess of emulsion is then removed from the cotton wool. It is at this point that the usefulness of Gamgee becomes apparent for the covering gauze adds to the strength of the material which can be rolled up and wrung out by hand. This must be done thoroughly until the cotton wool appears virtually dry and no more emulsion can be extracted. The sheet of cotton wool is left to dry off on a warm surface and when autoclaved is ready for use. For ease of handling it can be wrapped in cellophane or packed in a tin.

by elastoplast this should be used instead. The objective is as complete immobility as can be achieved and both the elastoplast and crepe are used to this end. Plaster of Paris should be used if it is felt that it will add significantly to the overall immobility of the grafted area.

There is no doubt that the pressure dressing method is at its most successful when a graft is used primarily. The pressure itself acts as a haemostatic factor preventing haematoma which might separate graft from bed. This is particularly true of the bolus part of the dressing for it is fitted to the graft with considerable accuracy.

It tends also to be most effective in the areas which can most easily be immobilised, for example the limbs and face. It might be argued that the face is mobile but the tie-over bolus, coupled in the early post-operative stages with the overall immobilising pressure of crepe and elastoplast, is enough to overcome major movements.

Pressure dressings tend to be used exclusively in the management of the whole skin graft. Such grafts are almost invariably used primarily and, fitted accurately with sutures to the defect, are scarcely candidates for the exposure method.

The problems of the pressure dressing method become more obvious applied to such areas as the neck and the groin, both extremely difficult to immobilise effectively, and the trunk where pressure as well as immobilisation is equally difficult to provide. It is in these areas that the pressure dressing method has really been found wanting. One approach is to use increasingly elaborate methods of immobilisation; the other, and it is the one increasingly being used, is to discard pressure dressings entirely and use exposed grafting.

EXPOSED GRAFTING

When the pressure dressing method was the only one in use it was recognised that certain areas were notoriously difficult to graft successfully and it was to solve the problems of grafting these areas that exposed grafting was developed. Its success in these situations has led to its invasion of previously undisputed pressure grafting territory.

The factor common to all the surfaces where it was first used was that they could not be immobilised. Even with the most elaborate methods of fixation and immobilisation the dressing tended to move to and fro, setting up shearing movements between graft and bed which prevented vascular link-up (Fig. 3.6). In those areas the pressure dressing, instead of being a means to the desired end of providing close, immobile contact, had become the means of preventing that end. Complete removal of the dressing eliminates these shearing strains at a single stroke and this fact forms the basis of the technique. The method relies on the natural fibrin adhesion between graft and bed—merely laid in position and protected from being rubbed off, the graft is allowed to lie until vascularisation and fixation have taken place in the usual way (Fig. 3.23).

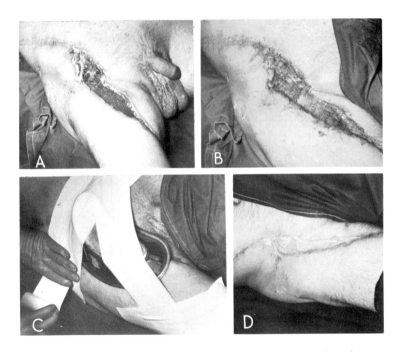

Fig. 3.23 Exposed grafting used in the treatment of a granulating surface of the groin. The raw area followed the flap necrosis which so often complicates radical groin dissection, in this instance an inguinopelvic lymph node clearance for metastatic squamous carcinoma. The granulating surface (A) is covered with a thin split-skin graft (B) and protected by the inverted kidney dish (C). (D) shows the end result.

It will be apparent that exposure has solved the problem of shearing movements but not the problems of haematoma and it is this factor which governs most of the practical details of the technique. Applied to the healthy granulating area problems of haemostasis do not arise and the method can work most effectively in such a situation. The post-surgical defect is more difficult and the method can then be used either **primarily, delayed** or **late**.

While it is possible to use **primary exposed grafting** the fact that pressure cannot be used once the graft has been applied means that haemostasis must be most rigorous. Though to be able to watch the graft does allow any little haematoma to be evacuated immediately by carefully snipping, the method is nonetheless not at its best used primarily.

Delayed exposed grafting is the alternative; in it the actual application of the graft is held over for a few days, the graft itself being stored meantime in the refrigerator (see p. 98). By waiting in this way complete haemostasis is assured and at the same time the wait is not so long that infection has a chance to develop. In the event the graft is applied when the surface looks healthy and free of clot. The interval is a variable one.

The surface can be left to granulate, and in certain circumstances this may be preferable, before the graft is applied. This is **late exposed grafting** and its practice does not differ in essence from exposed grafting of any granulating surface.

Exposed grafting does call for co-operation from the patient and so it must be used with discretion in children. The periods of least co-operation are during recovery from the anaesthetic and during transfer from theatre to bed. This is an added reason for using delayed grafting rather than primary grafting. It is usual to cut the graft at the time of the excisional procedure and store it in the refrigerator until it is required and can be applied with the patient awake and co-operative in bed.

The graft itself must be applied carefully; whether backed with tulle gras is a matter of personal preference. The tulle gras backing is convenient for handling but the graft tends to adapt itself more accurately to irregular surfaces minus the slightly rigid backing. The best of both worlds can be achieved by peeling the tulle gras off once the graft is in position.

The skin can be applied in a single sheet, or in more than one if the area is particularly big. Care should be taken to expel all air bubbles from under the graft which should be allowed to overlap the edge of the defect. It is quite remarkable how quickly the graft adheres firmly to its bed.

Protection can be improvised and need not be unduly elaborate. In fact it can be discarded altogether quite quickly if the patient is reasonably co-operative. If the area is small an inverted stainless steel bowl or kidney dish strapped over the defect is adequate; Kramer wire splinting is a useful and versatile material used in this context. Simple added fixation can be provided by micropore tape fixing the margins of the graft to the surrounding skin. If tape is used it should be left in place on the graft until it is well fixed in place. Attempts to peel it off are all too liable to pull the graft off its bed.

Using exposed grafting it naturally becomes possible to watch the graft vascularise. It is striking how speed of vascularisation appears to vary with the thickness of the graft. A factor in this of course may be the comparative opacity of the thicker graft which prevents the colour of the raw area from showing through but the development of pinkness is certainly strikingly slower in the thick graft.

There are many areas which can clearly be grafted successfully using either pressure or exposure. The technique chosen tends then to be a matter of personal preference, though in general exposed grafting is being increasingly used in many centres. Not least it can be a tremendous saver of operative time, saving as it does the time spent on suturing and application of dressing. It is worth trying when pressure methods have failed, and in the problem of the small granulating areas between previously applied stamps or sheets, those areas so troublesome and difficult to get either to heal or accept a graft using pressure methods.

GRAFTING GRANULATIONS

The skin graft can be applied in such a way that the entire surface is covered with the graft in the form of one or more large sheets. Alternatively, the graft may be applied in the form of strips or small stamps. Each of these strips or stamps applied to the granulating surface forms a focus from which epidermis spreads to cover the area between the individual stamps, the final healed surface being a mosaic of graft alternating with spread epidermis. Such a surface does tend to give a poor cosmetic result though the actual appearance in different patients shows wide and quite unpredictable variation. At the one extreme the spread epidermis is smooth and not unlike the stamps; at the other it becomes hypertrophic or even keloid. Initially redder, it usually pales to a colour more nearly matching the stamp over a period of months.

The spread epidermis is less stable than the stamp and in the lower limb, if support is not provided with elastic or crepe bandaging for a considerable period, small haemorrhagic blisters tend to form. Gradually it becomes more stable, stability and cosmetic improvement usually progressing together.

Sheets are less subject to these disadvantages and the trend has been towards an increasing use of them rather than stamps where ample skin is available (Fig. 3.24). Stamps are mainly justifiable where skin is in short supply or where fixation is difficult, as in

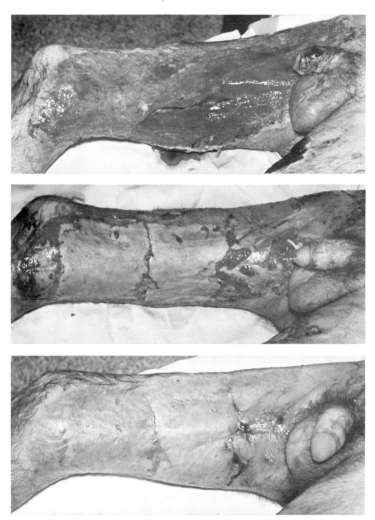

Fig. 3.24 The use of large sheet split-skin grafts in covering a granulating area of thigh.

perineum or axilla, when stamps are less likely to be dislodged than a sheet of skin which might become ruffled.

The mechanics of applying the graft are similar regardless of whether pressure or exposure is to be used. Spreading the graft on a sheet of tulle gras (Fig. 3.25) eases handling; tulle gras and graft can then be applied directly to the granulating area. The graft is not usually sutured in place, though in a difficult situation a few tacking sutures may help prevent it sliding off the granulations while the dressing is being applied. There is no question of using the sutures for a tie-over dressing for they would cut out very rapidly. In fact the use of sutures in such circumstances has largely been replaced by micropore tape which can be used to fix the graft to the surrounding skin.

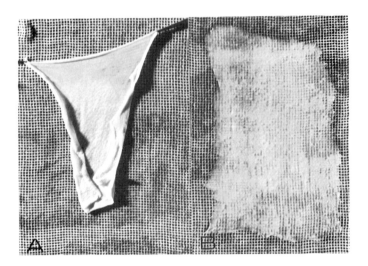

Fig. 3.25 The handling of a split-skin graft on tulle gras.
A   Laying the graft on the tulle gras which has been spread on a wooden board.
B   The graft spread on the tulle gras.

The recent development of **mesh grafting** has given a considerable boost to the use of the expanded graft, until then only possible by division into stamps. The graft, cut in the usual way, is passed through an instrument from which it emerges shredded into a regular meshwork of skin. Traction applied to the four corners of the graft expands the mesh giving an increase in area (Fig. 3.26). The advantage of the mesh graft over the stamp graft lies in the regularity of the mesh and the uniform distribution of the graft as a source of spread epidermis (Fig. 3.27). With the area between the strips so small the ultimate healing time becomes relatively short. As with stamps the final cosmetic result varies greatly and this is its main fault but in areas where cosmesis is a secondary consideration it does allow skin to be applied with success to surfaces where take would be regarded as moot using the other methods.

When pressure dressings are being used the graft and the dressing can readily be applied in theatre. Fixation of the graft is naturally much less secure than that provided by a tie-over dressing and it is

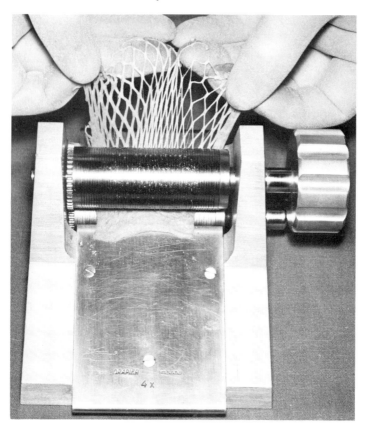

Fig. 3.26 Meshing a skin graft. The split-skin graft, fed between the rollers, emerges meshed so that, stretched, it can be expanded to cover a much larger area.

liable to slip during the first few turns of the bandage if these are not carefully applied. The outer dressing consists of the usual gauze, cotton wool, and crepe bandage or elastoplast. Bulk of dressing may be enough to produce immobility but plaster of Paris should always be used if need be to reinforce the dressings.

When exposure is being used it is better to wait until the patient is conscious and back in bed. The graft is then protected until it is well fixed.

Exposed grafting tends to be more effective when a single surface is being grafted; it is clearly impossible to use it if the area cannot be kept free of the bed clothes and this makes it inappropriate in most circumferential raw areas.

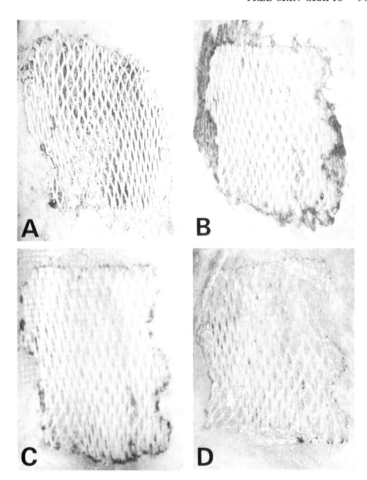

Fig. 3.27 The use of a mesh graft.

    A shows the mesh graft applied to a granulating area.

B and C show the intermediate stage of healing by epidermal spread from the graft, seen by the increased blurring of the outline of the mesh.

    D The healed result, showing how the background of the original mesh is still visible.

THE SEROMA

When a graft has been applied to a concave surface it sometimes, after it has become vascularised but before it has become firmly anchored to its bed, becomes detached from this bed over part of its area and tents across the concavity. This leaves a space underneath which fills with serum, creating a **seroma**. It tends to occur following the use of a pressure dressing and detachment takes place when pressure is removed a week after grafting. Aspiration of the serum is completely ineffective; the seroma rapidly reforms. While it is detached the graft remains surprisingly well vascularised from the surrounding attached graft.

Untreated, the graft proceeds to epithelialise on its deep surface from the cut ends of the pilosebaceous apparatus and eventually 'heals' completely. Since the graft cannot become re-attached once 'healing' has taken place treatment is a matter of some urgency.

Once it is recognised that the condition is due to contraction of the graft with resulting detachment and that the seroma is secondary to this, treatment is obvious. The graft must be cut open over the area of detachment in such a way that it lies completely and demonstrably quite freely on its bed. A cruciform cut may be needed before all tendency to tenting is corrected, for contraction of the graft has been in all axes. Treated without delay, these measures suffice but if several days have elapsed it must be assumed that some 'healing' has occurred and it is advisable to remove this epithelium by gently curetting the deep surface of the graft so that it can re-adhere. Alternatively, of course, the detached area of skin can be removed completely and a fresh graft applied.

STORAGE OF SKIN

By storage at a low temperature skin cut in excess of current requirements can be preserved viable for later use as needed. The current increase in the use of delayed exposed grafting has greatly increased the need for storage. Within the temperature range $0°$ C to $37°$ C the survival time of a stored graft is a function of its temperature and the lower the temperature the longer the survival time.

The experimental work which shows this has been done mainly with animal skin but enough is known of the behaviour of human skin similarly stored to make the results clinically applicable. For long survival Ringer's or Tyrode's solution should probably be used to keep the graft moist but normal saline works adequately. The graft is wrapped in gauze wet with the solution and placed in a sterile, sealed container. Unless specially long survival, e.g. up to 21 days, is needed, the storage temperature is not of paramount importance but it seems probable that $4°$ C is likely to give the best results.

LOCAL ANAESTHESIA FOR GRAFT-CUTTING

Formerly the use of local anaesthesia for graft cutting was restricted by the uneven surface which infiltration produced coupled with the large volume of anaesthetic agent needed. The use of hyaluronidase has removed these drawbacks and it is possible now to cut quite large grafts readily if the enzyme is added to the anaesthetic solution. The solution diffuses so rapidly that it is difficult to define exactly the area infiltrated and it is wise to outline the area to be anaesthetised with Bonney's Blue so that it can be systematically infiltrated. The exact amount of hyaluronidase which has to be used is not critical; 1500 i.u. added to 100 ml of anaesthetic solution will be found to work satisfactorily.

4

Skin flaps

A skin flap, in contradistinction to a free skin graft, retains a vascular attachment to the body at all times during transfer. It must therefore possess a vascular system, arterial, capillary and venous, capable of perfusing its tissues effectively throughout each stage of the transfer from donor to recipient site. The need for such a system means that most flaps must include both skin and underlying superficial fascia and the presence of such a system enables a flap to be transferred to an area whose blood supply would be inadequate to nourish a free skin graft.

In its simplest form a skin flap may be defined as a tongue of tissue which consists of skin plus a variable amount of underlying superficial fascia. It is transferred in order to reconstruct a **primary defect** and is **inset** into this defect (Fig. 4.1). Its transfer leaves a **secondary defect** and this is either closed by direct suture or covered with a free skin graft. (Fig. 4.1). When the flap is raised from the tissue immediately adjoining or very close to the primary defect it is called a **local flap**; when transfer of the flap involves moving tissue at a distance from the primary defect it is called a **distant flap**.

Some flaps, at the time of transfer, are reattached to the body over their entire area, and the proximal end of such a flap, where it becomes continuous with the adjacent skin, is referred to as its **base** (Fig. 4.2). With other flaps the **distal segment** alone of the flap is inset into the defect, its central segment and base remaining unattached. The base is then called the **pedicle** of the flap and the central segment is referred to as its **bridge segment** (Fig. 4.1). These two, pedicle and bridge segment, act as the carrier and provide the channel of blood supply to the distal segment. Once the distal segment is established in its new site, which usually takes three weeks, the bridge segment is divided and either returned to its original site or discarded, depending on the local situation. Insetting of the distal segment is then completed.

The pedicle of a skin flap usually consists, like the rest of the flap,

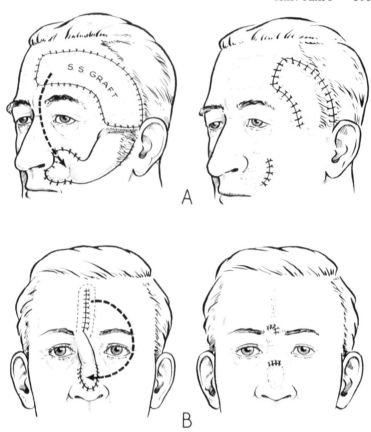

Fig. 4.1 Examples of skin flap transfers. In both a *single pedicled* flap has been used to reconstruct the *primary defect* and the *distal segment* has been *inset* into it. The *secondary defect* has been closed by split-skin graft in A, by direct suture in B. Once the distal segment has been established in its new site the *bridge segment* has been returned to its original position in A, discarded in B. Insetting of the distal segment has then been completed.

of skin and subcutaneous tissue but it is occasionally reduced to its subcutaneous component. In such circumstances it is the distal segment with a full complement of skin and subcutaneous tissue which is transferred, as an **island flap** (Fig. 8.3).

When a local flap is transferred, movement usually takes the form of **rotation** or **transposition**. The name is then applied to the flap (Fig. 4.2).

When a distant flap is transferred it is raised prior to its transfer either with a **single pedicle**, as a tongue of tissue (Fig. 4.3), or **bipedicled,** as a strap of tissue with a pedicle at each end (Fig. 4.3).

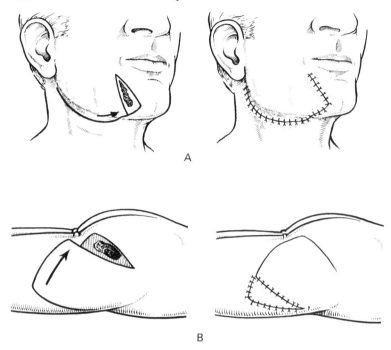

Fig. 4.2 Examples of *local flaps*. In both the flap is elevated as far as its *base*. In A movement to cover the primary defect is by *rotation*, in B by *transposition*. In A there is no secondary defect, in B the secondary defect is split-skin grafted.

Whenever possible the bridge segment of a flap is **tubed** in order to eliminate unnecessary raw surface and reduce sepsis. A bipedicled flap, tubed in this way, is called a **tube pedicle**.

A distant flap can be transferred to its destination in several ways. It can be **directly applied** to the primary defect. It may be attached to a **carrier**, usually the wrist, on which it is conveyed to its destination (Fig. 4.4). The wrist is selected as a carrier because its reach makes it possible for the flap to leap-frog a considerable distance in one step. The flap may also be swung on its pedicle and **waltzed** to its destination (Fig. 4.4). This method tends to be used only when the distance between the flap and the primary defect is not great and a single waltzing movement completes the transfer.

It is sometimes felt that the blood supply of a flap would not be adequate for its survival if it were raised and transferred straight-away. Its vascular efficiency can be improved by surgically outlining the flap before its actual transfer and such outlining is called a **delay**. Other circumstances arise during flap transfer when it is also judged

Bipedicled flap converted
into tube pedicle

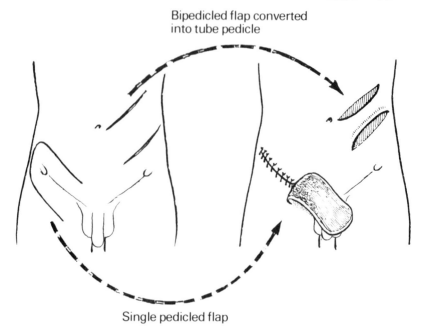

Single pedicled flap

Fig. 4.3 Raising *distant flaps* on the abdomen. The single pedicled flap was raised on groin, the *bipedicled flap* has been raised, its secondary defect being split-skin grafted and converted into a *tube pedicle*.

necessary to augment the blood supply of the flap by a surgical procedure and the term is applied to these procedures also.

Most local flaps have an axis around which they rotate or are transposed and this is called the **pivot point** of the flap (Fig. 4.29). During design it is from the pivot point that measurements are made to ensure that the geometry of the flap will allow it to achieve its transfer. When a local flap is jumping over intact tissue and also with distant flaps generally an alternative technique, planning in reverse, is used, but its purpose is the same.

Flaps vary greatly in their robustness, reserve of safety, ease of execution, time taken to complete and convenience generally. The importance of these factors in selecting the flap to use in specific clinical situations is being increasingly appreciated and acted upon. The most striking example of this has been the downgrading in importance and usage generally of the tube pedicle and certain direct flaps.

The tube pedicle was historically an extremely significant development in plastic surgery and there is still something of a mystique associated with it. Although it still has its uses it has been superseded in virtually every sphere where it was at one time pre-eminent.

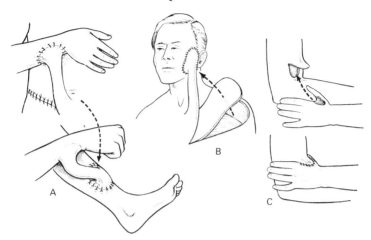

Fig. 4.4 Examples of techniques of transfer of distant flaps. In A, a single pedicled flap has been raised, with closure of the secondary defect by direct suture. Its distal end has been attached to a *wrist carrier* on which it has been conveyed to its destination on the leg. In B, a single pedicled flap raised on the chest has been *waltzed* to its destination on the face. In C, a single pedicled flap has been raised on the upper arm and *directly applied* to the primary defect of the 1st web, the hand with its defect having been brought to the flap so that transfer can take place.

It takes too long to complete its transfer, it is too prone to vascular complications, and all too often, particularly in transfer to the lower limb, it places too heavy demands on the tolerance of the patient. Experienced plastic surgeons tend now to use it only as a last resort.

Some of the adverse factors relating to the tube pedicle apply with equal and even greater force to certain direct flaps, particularly the cross-leg flap (p. 156), and for similar reasons the plastic surgeon with experience will go to considerable lengths to avoid using them because they are so demanding on both patient and surgeon and have such an inadequate safety factor of vascular reserve.

Problems of blood supply dominate all aspects of flap transfer. The surgeon soon becomes aware that adequate blood flow with effective tissue perfusion is a crucial factor at every stage of the transfer. Within the limits imposed by the demands of circulation and consequent flap viability the surgeon constantly tries to achieve the most advantageous geometry possible for his flap. Skill in the design and use of flaps is very much a matter of balancing the demands of flap blood supply against those of flap geometry.

For a flap to be long in relation to its breadth is always the wish of the surgeon. It makes the transfer technically easier, reducing the need for ultra-care in planning and rigid post-operative immobilisation.

Two flap types can be distinguished according to their vascular characteristics and behaviour patterns, each with a distinctive geometry imposed by its vascular anatomy, those with an *axial pattern* and those with a *random pattern* of blood vessels.

Axial pattern flap (Fig. 4.5). This is a single pedicled flap which has a pre-existing anatomically recognised arteriovenous system running along its long axis. The system running along its length makes it possible to construct the flap at least as long as the territory of its axial artery with minimal regard for considerations of breadth.

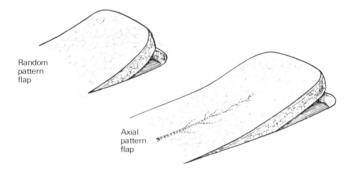

Random pattern flap

Axial pattern flap

Fig. 4.5 Stylised versions of *random* and *axial pattern flaps*. For simplicity only the axial artery is shown but an equally effective axial venous system is also present in practice. The random flap shows the limitation of length-breadth ratio to approximately 1:1. The length of the axial flap is governed by the territory of the axial vessels though it has been found that the flap found safe in practice extends beyond the territory as shown. This distal segment can be viewed as random on the end of the axial segment.

Random pattern flap (Fig. 4.5). This is a flap in which the pattern of arteries and veins lacks sufficient axial bias to be of any practical use. Because of the random nature of its vascular pattern such a flap is subject to fairly stringent limitations in dimensions, particularly in its permissible length-breadth ratio. These limitations have long been recognised and accepted by surgeons experienced in the use of such flaps.

The concept of length-breadth ratio as a limiting factor is not an absolutely precise concept and the stringency with which it has to be applied varies depending on the vascularity of the skin area under consideration, particularly the richness of its subdermal plexus. Facial skin for example is extremely vascular and it is possible as a result to relax length-breadth restrictions considerably. It is in the trunk and limbs that the restrictions have to be applied much more rigidly.

However imprecise the length-breadth ratio concept and however many exceptions there may be in the head and neck there are no other criteria which are remotely comparable in effectiveness. Outside the head and neck a random pattern flap with a length-breadth greater than 1:1 is likely to suffer from vascular inadequacy unless steps are taken to enhance its vascular efficiency, by a delay for example, and allow it to be constructed longer than it is broad.

Axial pattern flaps have significant advantages over random pattern flaps. The relative freedom from dimensional restrictions, particularly in the ratio of length to breadth, makes them easier and safer to transfer with less need for ultra-care in planning. The length of the flap reduces the need for rigid immobilisation post-operatively. The great increase in vascular reserve makes the flap safer, more robust and better able to cope with adverse circumstances. It is also possible to raise such a flap, convert it into a tube and carry out the first stage of its transfer in a single stage, eliminating the preliminary six weeks maturation required of the classic tube pedicle.

VASCULAR ASPECTS OF FLAPS

Blood supply governs all flap practice and a clear understanding of this aspect will explain much which would otherwise be inexplicable in the construction and transfer of individual flaps, whether they are axial or random in type.

VASCULAR ADJUSTMENTS

Unless a flap has been specifically designed to include in its substance a pre-existing anatomically recognised arteriovenous system the plastic surgeon designs it on the assumption that its blood vessels lack sufficient bias in direction to influence its design significantly. Such a flap differs from the surrounding skin in that its quota of arteries and veins is strictly limited. This can be seen if one considers the theoretical situation of a square flap with vascular pattern distributed equally on each side and its deep surface. Raising such flap to leave it attached by one side alone reduces its vascular capacity to one-fifth, and though such a theoretical distribution of blood vessels does not hold in practice the principle of reduction of vascular capacity does.

If, however, it were possible to cut off the other four vascular attachments gradually it would be found that the pattern of the flap had adjusted itself so that its capacity and reserve remained almost normal. Little is known of the mechanics of these changes but a more efficient vascular pattern is presumably produced. Structurally there appears to be an axial reorientation of the larger blood vessels with an increase in number and calibre.

The vessels of the flap are of course totally denervated by the elevation. The normal skin colour indicates that they are not dilated; they develop an autonomous state of tone and are capable in appropriate circumstances of producing the pattern of dilatation appropriate to reactive hyperaemia and acute inflammation.

Pattern changes are less necessary when an axial arteriovenous system is already present if the flap being raised lies within the territory supplied by the system. It has been found in practice, however, that axial pattern flaps are regularly safely raised which extend beyond the demonstrated territory of their axial arterio-venous system. The area outwith the territory found safe approxi-mates to a square. It can be viewed as being in the nature of a 'random pattern flap' on the end of the true axial pattern flap.

VASCULAR INADEQUACY

When a random pattern flap is showing signs of vascular inadequacy the difficulty in most cases is not the getting of blood into the flap but getting the blood which is in, out. It is 'circulation' which is the problem. To lose a flap because of pure arterial insufficiency is rare; to lose part of all of it because of venous insufficiency is all too common. Several factors play a part singly or together in creating embarrassment of the circulation.

Mechanical tension and **kinking** of the flap are two of the more frequent causes. When a flap is being transferred it must not be sutured under greater than normal tension; tension should rather be less than normal. Kinking of a flap often indicates the presence of a shearing strain on its pedicle to the detriment of the circulation.

With venous pressure lower than arterial it is venous outflow which is impaired initially in most instances giving the flap a congested appearance. Kinking tends to be most serious when the flap lacks flexibility and it is always aggravated by any factors which increase tissue turgor.

Transient mild **oedema** is common even in the flap progressing favourably. It increases over the first 24 to 36 hours, remains for a further 2 to 3 days and then settles, fine wrinkling of the shiny oedematous skin being the first sign of its passing as the circulation becomes more efficient. Oedema of course adds to tissue turgor, changing skin previously lax and wrinkled into skin shiny and swollen, enhancing the ill effects of tension and kinking.

Inflammation in a flap is a potent cause of circulatory inadequacy. The vascular reserve of a flap is never normal and while it may be adequate to cope with ordinary metabolic needs the added burden of an inflammatory reaction must always be an embarrassment. The soil rather than the seed is the critical factor and infection which would be of minor significance elsewhere can produce necrosis of quite disastrous extent in a flap. When inflammatory oedema develops, tension becomes an added factor in causing the necrosis to spread.

These factors have been discussed separately but in practice they seldom act singly. One factor may initiate the vicious circle but rapidly the others come into action to aggravate the cycle schematically indicated in Figure 4.6.

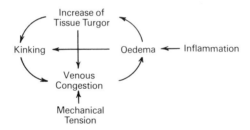

Fig. 4.6 The vicious circle of circulatory embarrassment in a flap.

The axial pattern flap has such a built-in reserve of capacity that these factors tend to have less of an embarrassing effect on the circulation. In particular the presence of an efficient venous pattern has the effect of making oedema of a flap, even as a transient phenomenon, very uncommon indeed. In practice steps are naturally taken to avoid these factors just as in random pattern flaps, but axial pattern flaps are better able to cope with their adverse effects.

The difference in the circulatory dynamics of the two flap types is strikingly shown by the skin colour. The colour of the healthy random pattern flap is pink, blanching on pressure with return of skin colour as quickly as in the surrounding skin. The healthy axial pattern flap is usually deathly white with virtually no circulation apparent in the skin at all and is taken to indicate an efficient venous system with rapid flow through. It is an appearance alarming to the inexperienced.

FLAP NECROSIS

In a random pattern flap developing necrosis presents clinically with the skin acutely congested, cyanosed, blanching momentarily on pressure, but with vessels rapidly filling again; the vascular bed is dilated and largely stagnant. As the condition progresses, blanching on pressure becomes less and less definite until there is clearly no active circulation. The cyanosis remains and takes on a violaceous tint. Histologically there is gross extravasation of blood. Blistering of the skin with serum, or blood-filled blebs, usually develops. When the blister skin is removed, the underlying skin is moist, cyanosed and without demonstrable circulation. Although the development of such blisters indicates that some circulation is still present it also implies that the onset of necrosis is virtually inevitable and imminent. At this point the margin of the affected area is seldom well demarcated and the process tends to spread for the reasons already indicated. The final area of necrosis is often more extensive than appearances at the onset might have suggested. This is so because the process will not halt until a skin area has been reached whose vascular capacity is able to cope not merely with ordinary meetabolic needs, but also with the added vascular burden of the adjacent necrosis and any superadded infection. When the process eventually does stop spreading a good line of demarcation is present with, just proximal to it, a zone of inflammation well sustained from a vascular viewpoint. The whole picture is an acute one, settled one way or the other in 1 to 2 days.

In the axial pattern flap the sequence is quite different. The vascular physiopathology underlying the clinical events is not fully understood. It takes several days to develop fully and during this period it is difficult to be sure whether the flap is going to recover or not. Instead of the intense pallor indicating a healthy flap, the area of concern is slightly cyanosed with what appears to be a sluggish circulation. The signs are not gross and can easily be missed iin the early stages. For several days the appearance remains virtually unchanged, transient improvement often occurring temporarily, until finally necrosis does become definite. The slow way in which the whole sequence evolves gives time for some revascularisation of the margin of the flap to occur from the surrounding tissues so that the final area of necrosis instead of being the entire distal flap is often an island in its centre.

Once seen, the premonitory slight cyanotic colouration, as opposed to the healthy pallor, is easily recognised again and its appearance usually means inevitable necrosis, though several days may elapse before it is acknowledged as such.

PREVENTION OF FLAP NECROSIS

Steps can be taken at all stages to prevent flap necrosis in the design of the flap, by enhancing its vascular efficiency and by care during and after transfer.

Design of the flap

In the random pattern flap this involves such factors as the length-breadth ratio, the intrinsic vascular pattern of the flap, its anatomical situation, etc., and the problems will be discussed as they relate to the planning of each kind of flap. *The design should always allow for the normal increase in tension which the phase of oedema creates.* In the axial pattern flap, design is more concerned with ensuring that the flap includes its axial arteriovenous system and does not extend beyond its recognised safe length.

When a flap is required which does extend beyond the known safe length it is necessary to make sure that the extension is capable of surviving based on the blood supply of the axial pattern element. This involves enhancing its vascular efficiency and the technique is also used to increase the safe length of random pattern flaps.

Enhancement of vascular efficiency

Where an axial arteriovenous system already exists no steps are required to enhance vascular efficiency unless the flap being raised is extending beyond its accepted safe length. Where such a system is not already present, as in the case of a random pattern flap, it is possible to enhance the vascular efficiency of the flap by the use of a **delay**. This manoeuvre permits the use of a greater length-breadth ratio than would be possible without it.

An incision is made along the line across which the surgeon wishes to cut off the blood supply, the blood vessels crossing the line are divided, ligated if need be, and the wound is resutured and allowed to heal (Fig. 4.7). This only divides marginal vessels and to cut off the blood supply entering the deep surface the flap must be elevated and the entering vessels divided and ligated before returning the flap to its original position. In a difficult situation the flap can be delayed in stages. Such vascular link-up as may occur during healing of the incision is not enough to prevent the redeployment of blood vessels which results.

These steps restrict the flap to the blood vessels on which it will have to rely at the time of the actual transfer without adding the strain of the transfer itself and 'train' it to rely on these vessels, probably by inducing in them a degree of axial re-orientation.

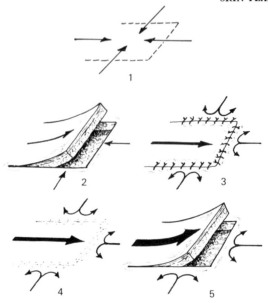

Fig. 4.7 The delay, showing in diagrammatic fashion its effect on the blood supply of the flap. The flap outlined (1) with its blood supply coming from all directions is raised (2) cutting off all blood vessels other than those entering and leaving its base. The flap is sutured back in position and 10–14 days later raised for transfer. During this time (3, 4) the blood supply remains restricted to that through the base and this supply increases in efficiency to nourish the flap during actual transfer (5). *For clarity the blood supply entering the deep surface of the flap has been omitted.*

When a delay is used to extend an axial pattern flap beyond its accepted safe length a similar technique is employed, raising the extension, in stages if necessary, so that its sole attachment is to the distal end of the axial pattern flap. The axial pattern flap, together with its extension is then transferred in the usual way. In such circumstances the added segment is described as having been **delayed** on to the end of the parent flap.

How soon the delay can be assumed to have achieved its purpose has never been properly worked out experimentally and the time is dictated by the healing of the incision. The next stage is proceeded with when the delay has healed, usually in 7 to 10 days (Fig. 4.8).

The delay is a double-edged weapon capable of operating against as well as for the surgeon. This is true especially of the delay involving elevation for, no matter how delicate the technique, reaction of the separated surfaces is always produced. Excision of this indurated surface when the flap is actually transferred does not altogether eliminate the zone of reaction and its presence undoubtedly reduces the flexibility of the flap, making kinking both more

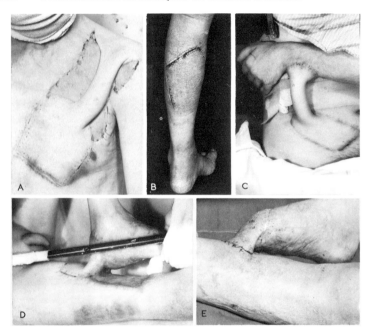

Fig. 4.8 Examples of surgical delays.
A 'Pancake' flap delayed on to one end of an acromiopectoral tube pedicle used to repair radionecrotic ulcer of chin shown in Figure 6.6B.
B Delay of cross-leg flap. Subsequent stages shown in E and Figure 4.42A.
C Lengthening an abdominal tube pedicle by delay.
D Delay of the segment of the cross-thigh flap (see Fig. 4.42D) planned in Figure 4.20, which was intended to cover the heel of the foot.
E Delay of cross-leg flap (see B and Fig. 4.42A) prior to detaching and inserting the flap.

likely and more serious. It is desirable to reduce reaction to an absolute minimum by using planes of cleavage. Not merely does this reduce the overall amount of reaction but the reaction itself tends to be restricted to the cleavage plane. Resection of this layer at the time of actual transfer of the flap largely restores its original flexibility. In the limb this is at the junction of superficial and deep fascia, in the abdomen at the junction of superficial fascia and aponeurosis. In the chest and back no real plane exists, but the best substitute is close to muscle. In the forehead and scalp the problem does not arise since a delay need never include elevation, blood supply being for practical purposes entirely marginal and with no deep connections.

Haematoma too adds to the reaction and should be avoided by scrupulous haemostasis. A carefully applied pressure dressing post-operatively will prevent the accumulation of fluid under a flap though a balance between too little pressure which allows fluid to gather and too much which causes ischaemic necrosis is not always easy to achieve.

Care during and after transfer

It is after transfer particularly that skilled and experienced nursing can be invaluable not merely in preventing trouble through careful positioning of the patient but in recognising the danger signals of circulatory embarrassment early while they are still readily reversible and before the inexorable sequence which leads to necrosis has begun in real earnest. The position of the recently attached flap or tube must also be checked frequently. Kinking for even a brief period can have a disastrous effect on its already taxed venous drainage and the proper position when the patient is stirring in his own bed may be quite different from that when he was quietly anaesthetised on the operating table. It is at this time too that a good nurse can provide the encouragement so necessary to a patient during the early hours and days of what for him may be a most uncomfortable position.

There are several ways however in which the surgeon can anticipate and prevent the potential troubles which can arise post-operatively.

Haemostasis. A developing haematoma is prone to initiate the increase of tension which starts the cycle of events already described. Haemostasis is easier to achieve if planes of cleavage are used, for the vessels crossing are large and few and are readily ligated. A previous delay tends to obscure these and a diffuse ooze is more common.

The way in which the flap itself is handled post-operatively can also be very significant. The usual alternatives are the pressure dressing or exposure with or without suction. With the increased use of suction the pressure dressing is deservedly losing its popularity. It is difficult to apply uniformly and its correct level is very much a hit or miss. It also makes hour to hour monitoring of the vascular state of the flap impossible. Exposure permits continuous assessment and, coupled with suction, it is probably more effective in preventing the development of disastrous haematoma. The minor ooze it can certainly cope with. Nevertheless the flap must still be watched carefully and if the tell-tale increase in swelling that spells haematoma cannot be controlled by suction the flap must be elevated and haemostasis achieved when the clot has been evacuated.

Control of sepsis. Infection as a factor operates at all stages and, with the sole exception of head and neck flaps, all skin surfaces are best healed before the next stage of the transfer is contemplated. Skin preparation must be scrupulous and though asepsis is often difficult to achieve at every stage of the various operations involved in the transfer, it must be realised that each break in technique does endanger the procedure. Planning at each stage to avoid raw surfaces is important and this topic is discussed on page 120. Measures to prevent haematoma aid also in the control of sepsis.

Many measures have been recommended in managing the flap showing signs of serious circulatory embarrassment, each with its own advocates but each lacking proper clinical controls and with more than a spice of wishful thinking. Cooling of the flap with the aim of reducing its metabolic rate, the use of low molecular dextran, and even hyperbaric oxygen have all been suggested, with more faith than observed fact to support them.

The use of intermittent and continuous pressure have both been advocated with the object of forcing the blood out into the veins by increasing the general pressure on the flap; in effect to provide an alternative peripheral resistance to the atonic, dilated local capillary bed of the flap suffering from vascular insufficiency. In theory, the optimum pressure should be just below capillary pressure. Critical assessment of either of these pressure methods is clearly impossible since there is no way of knowing what might have happened had other management methods been used.

On the other hand, the interference of gentle massage to try to keep the circulation going, inspection, etc., do more harm than good. They produce local hyperaemia in normal tissues and this is exactly what one wishes to avoid in a flap. It may well be that much of any success achieved by pressure techniques results from the rest which the flap is allowed. Neither intermittent nor continuous pressure methods have achieved much popularity.

To return the flap to its donor site until it has recovered has certain theoretical attractions but in practice the decision is apt to be delayed beyond the point of no return in viability of the flap. Depending on the reason for using the flap in the first place it may, in fact, prove more disastrous to return it than to leave it and await the outcome.

All in all, prevention by care in planning, execution and after care are preferable to the uncertainties of treating incipient flap necrosis.

TREATMENT OF FLAP NECROSIS

It will be apparent that there is a limit to what can be done to save a flap in danger of necrosing, but once necrosis is considered inevitable or is actually present the very presence of necrotic tissue inviting superadded infection tends to spread the process and the surgeon may make the bold decision to detach the flap, excise the dying segment, and re-inset it in the hope that removal of the necrotic focus will give the flap a fresh start. His problem is then to decide where the line of excision should be, and a good indication of the viability of a flap margin is the state of dermal bleeding, its colour and quantity.

Such a drastic course is only possible if the flap has been planned with a considerable margin of safety and failing this, a conservative policy must be pursued, awaiting slough demarcation and separation. When the resulting surface is favourable a split-skin graft may be applied but the disastrous effect of infection and fibrosis on the vascular attachment must be recognised and each subsequent step requires redoubled care, and the use of delays, etc. It is unfortunately true that a disaster of this sort during a flap transfer makes subsequent similar disasters much more probable.

TECHNIQUES USED IN FLAP PRACTICE

Certain techniques are common to the transfer of virtually all skin flaps and it is convenient to consider them collectively before discussing how they are applied in practice to the various flaps, local and distant, axial and random.

Raising a Flap

The standard flap is normally raised in the plane of surgical cleavage (Fig. 4.9).

On the trunk and limbs this plane is between superficial fascia and muscle, aponeurosis or deep fascia; on the scalp it is between galea aponeurotica and pericranium. In both of these areas the vessels which cross the plane of surgical cleavage are few and readily picked up for ligation or largely absent and this makes the raising of a flap technically much easier. The use of this plane also leaves a bed which takes a free skin graft readily.

The face has no comparable plane and one has to be artificially created when a flap is being raised. The level chosen is in the fat just deep to the dermis, leaving the flap with the beneficial effect of the richly vascular subdermal plexus of facial skin but without disturbing the facial nerve or muscles.

The area over which the flap is raised varies with the task it is required to perform. In general it should be raised over at least the entire area of skin ultimately to be transferred but the demands of

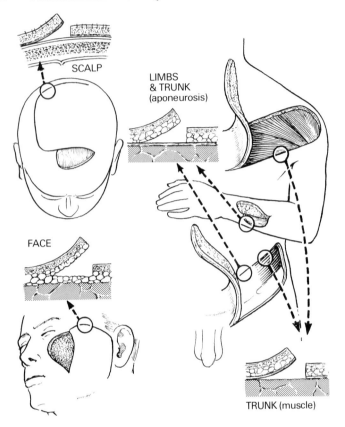

Fig. 4.9 The levels at which flaps are normally raised; in the scalp, face, limbs and trunk. Note the difference in level on the trunk depending on whether the flap is raised over muscle or aponeurosis.

the transfer may require its being raised considerably further, to provide a bridge segment and pedicle for example.

Raised in this way the flap is often thicker than is desirable and a certain amount of thinning may be necessary. The need for thinning, the method of thinning and the amount which is safe, vary with the type of flap and its site.

For reasons too obvious to need stressing, excessively fat patients make bad subjects for flaps. This applies with even greater force when one of their more adipose areas is the donor site of the flap. Even in ordinary circumstances but much more so when it is present in excess, fat is not a surgically rewarding tissue to work with. Fat necrosis is always a potential hazard and even in a mild form it is capable of triggering off a disastrous inflammatory episode.

Thinning a flap

The **face** is an extremely vascular site with a highly developed subdermal circulation and certain of the flaps raised in this site are thinned considerably. In practice it is rarely necessary to thin the large flaps, the initial level approximating usually to the final level. It is the smaller flaps which are more often thinned and this can safely be quite drastic, leaving the flap with virtually no fat but relying largely on its subdermal circulation.

Scalp flaps are raised at the subgaleal level and the physical characters of scalp are such that thinning is rarely, if ever, carried out.

On the **limbs**, flaps seldom require to be thinned because the layer of subcutaneous fat is not thick enough to warrant it.

On the **trunk**, which provides the source for most of the larger flaps, the factors which determine whether a flap is thinned are more complex. When thinning is required it is carried out either in order to match the thickness of the defect or to allow the flap to be tubed without undue tension and at the same time retain reasonable flexibility of its bridge segment.

Even if formal thinning is not carried out, trimming of the fat along the margin of the flap is desirable as a rule (Fig. 4.10). As usually raised, lobules of fat tend to bulge over the skin edge of the flap and their presence there makes a neat suture line, marginal or along the tubing seam, difficult to achieve because of the little fat herniations which bulge between the individual sutures. It is this marginal fat which can safely be trimmed back without detriment to the blood supply of the flap.

It is also safer to thin a random pattern flap to a thickness which will allow it to be tubed without tension than leave it thicker but tubed only with difficulty. The larger blood vessels fortunately run fairly superficial in the fascia and there is also evidence that the subdermal plexus makes a greater contribution to the vascular efficiency of a flap than has been generally appreciated. The hand holding the flap for thinning should be used to judge the amount required. Touch gives a much more accurate measure than vision alone and thinning is carried out uniformly over the entire surface (Fig. 4.10).

In the case of an axial pattern flap on the trunk the problem varies with the site of the flap and the sex of the patient. In the male the chest and upper abdomen are not particularly adipose and thinning is not often needed. Vigorous trimming of the marginal fat may suffice. The presence of the breast in the female complicates matters when the flap encroaches upon it, particularly where the breast is

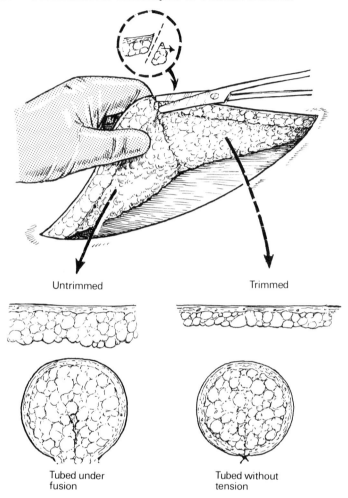

Untrimmed

Trimmed

Tubed under
fusion

Tubed without
tension

Fig. 4.10 Thinning a random flap, including trimming of the margins to allow the flap to be tubed without tension.

large and pendulous. The surgeon should have no hesitation about thinning the flap to make its overall thickness correspond to that of the part of the flap outwith the margin of the breast. Thinning is usually being carried out to allow tubing and need only be rigorous enough for this purpose.

The problem of thinning is less easily solved when the flap is being raised from the lower abdomen and groin. This is a notoriously fat site in many adults and the presence of fat in excess may indeed be a valid reason for selecting an alternative site when a flap is being planned.

The axial pattern flaps in the groin area each contain a single axial artery. Near its source from the femoral artery this vessel is running deep in the superficial fascia, becoming more superficial as it passes distally. Towards the distal end of each flap and plexus which forms the basis of its vascular supply is superficial in the fascia. Making use of this fact experienced surgeons have found it safe to thin the distal part of such flaps considerably. Thinning must of course be done with care, preferably with magnification, and probably not by the inexeperienced surgeon. The lobules of fat are individually dissected off the flap without disturbing the plexus. Increasing care is required with passage proximally to ensure that the axial system is not damaged. Thinning of this part of the flap is less often required in any case, the proximal segment usually acting as the bridge segment and not part of the ultimately transferred tissue. Its thinness is important only in allowing it to be tubed.

Avoidance of infection

The blood supply of many flaps is less than optimal and unnecessary demands upon it are undesirable. A particularly disastrous demand which can be added to the normal load is that of an inflammatory reaction. For this reason every precaution is taken to avoid infection during the transfer of a flap. Apart from the obvious use of an aseptic technique at operation and subsequent dressings, two steps are normally taken to avoid infection. These are **prevention of haematoma** and **avoidance of raw areas**.

Prevention of haematoma. Assuming careful haemostasis at operation the most effective measure which can be taken postoperatively to prevent haematoma is the use of suction. The larger the area of the surfaces apposed by the transfer of the flap the greater the need of suction drainage to ensure that the surfaces are not separated by haematoma but adhere to one another quickly.

Various commercial suction drains are available but my own preference is for a wide bore catheter with additional openings cut. The catheter can be placed under the flap, either through the marginal suture line or via an independent stab incision. If the bridge segment of the flap has been tubed the catheter can be inserted along its length to lie beneath the distal end of the flap (Fig. 4.11).

Although present discussion concerns haematoma in relation to infection it may be mentioned also that its occurrence has the further adverse effect of preventing vascular link-up between flap and bed. The importance of rapid and effective adhesion of a flap to its bed should not be underestimated both in reducing the chances of

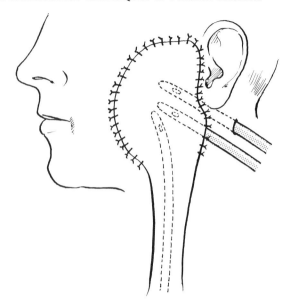

Fig. 4.11 The various ways in which suction can be used to achieve deep adhesion of the distal end of a flap, via a separate incision, using the marginal suture line, or along the length of the tubed bridge segment.

serious infection and in encouraging the development of a good vascular attachment. To achieve this suction is invaluable.

Avoidance of raw areas. Raw surfaces with their potential for infection are eliminated either by **direct closure** or by **grafting**.

Direct closure is used in various ways. The secondary defect may be closed by direct suture but as a rule this is possible only in the face where the skin is often lax and available for closure without tension. Skin is less readily available elsewhere on the body surface and direct suture of secondary defects is rarely possible.

The flap itself is often closed over part of its length by tubing its bridge segment when one exists (Fig. 4.12). Outside the face and scalp tubing is carried out whenever possible; in the face and scalp the characteristics of the tissues involved and the relative narrowness of the flap often makes tubing physically impossible. Partial tubing by loosely folding the flap and grafting its bridge segment are used when possible if the raw surface is large in area. Fortunately the vascular reserve of most facial flaps allows them to cope with the load of a raw surface and infection from this source is rare.

If it is proposed to tube a flap it may be desirable to tattoo matching points along its margins with Bonney's Blue, for use once the flap has been raised. With these matching points approximated

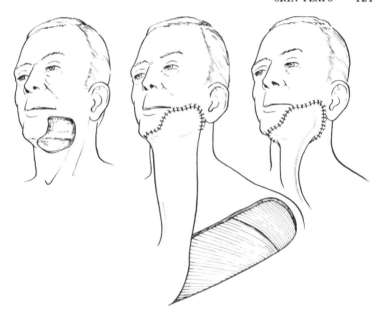

Fig. 4.12 Avoidance of raw surface by tubing the bridge segment of a flap. In this way the entire raw area on the deep surface of the flap is eliminated.

using interrupted sutures so that tension is distributed correctly, a continuous 'over and over' suture can be used between to close the seam.

When the secondary defect is being grafted tension develops as tubing proceeds towards the base of the flap. As soon as there is any suggestion of difficulty in bringing the skin edges together tubing should be stopped. When the secondary defect is being closed by direct suture such tension does not develop, the seaming suture line of the tube and the suture line of the secondary defect meeting at the base of the tube. There a modified three point suture can be used to close the junction point.

Skin grafting is most frequently used to close the secondary defect created by the raising of the flap. The grafting method used depends on whether or not the flap in its raised position remains directly overlying the secondary defect or not. When the flap overlies the defect the use of a tie-over bolus pressure dressing is unavoidable. When the secondary defect is not covered by the flap postoperatively, delayed exposed grafting becomes possible, and is frequently preferable.

When a tie-over bolus pressure dressing is being used under a tubed flap it must be applied with considerable care, particularly near the base of the flap to get the necessary immobilisation and approximation of the graft without being bulky enough to embarrass the circulation of the flap.

It may not be possible to tube the bridge segment of a flap because it is too short, as in the case of most direct flaps and instead its raw surface is skin grafted. The split-skin graft used to cover the secondary defect is made longer and carried on to the flap so that its raw surface is covered with skin (Fig. 4.13). In the case of a direct flap the secondary defect is almost invariably grafted using the pressure bolus method and it is important to make sure that the pressure applied to the graft does not extend on to the bridge segment to the detriment of its blood supply.

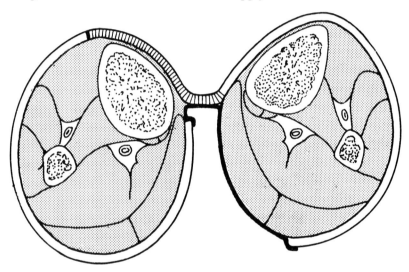

Fig. 4.13 Avoidance of raw surface during transfer of a direct flap, by extending the split-skin graft used to cover the secondary defect to line the short bridge segment of the flap.

Mechanisms of flap transfer (Fig. 4.14)

When a single pedicle flap is raised and tubed in preparation for transfer, tubing is stopped towards its distal end leaving an approximately circular raw surface. When a tube pedicle is detached at one end in preparation for reattachment elsewhere, a similarly circular raw surface is produced on the flap. In both instances the surgeon uses this raw surface to reattach the flap in its new site. In the new site he creates a comparably shaped raw surface. The two raw surfaces are apposed one to the other and since they correspond in shape and size, closure of the skin edges eliminates both.

When the flap is being transferred on a carrier the reception raw surface is made on the wrist; if the flap is being waltzed, the site of the raw surface is positioned in accordance with the overall design of the transfer (p. 125). In either event the circular raw surface is created by elevating a semicircular trap-door of skin and superficial fascia. The circular shape gives a maximum of raw surface contact with a consequent beneficial effect on the speed and effectiveness of the vascular link-up.

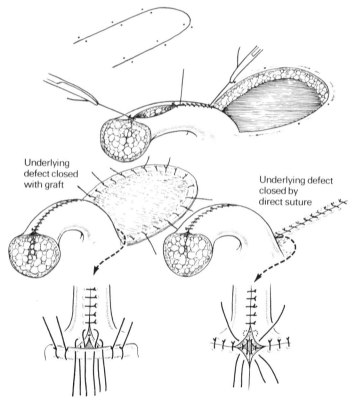

Underlying defect closed with graft

Underlying defect closed by direct suture

Fig. 4.14 Raising and tubing a single pedicled flap in preparation for transfer, showing steps in closing the secondary defect by split-skin graft and by direct suture.

Design of the trap-door. While in theory the trap-door should have the same width, etc., as the flap it is wise in practice to allow for shrinkage of the flap. The trap-door is best made a little smaller than the flap dimensions might indicate to positively eliminate flap tension. The correct size for the trap-door can be ascertained easily by making a blood-stained imprint of the raw surface of the flap at the site of the planned attachment.

The siting of the trap-door depends on whether transfer is by **carrier** or **waltzing**.

Carrier (Fig. 4.15). The site will be the ulnar or radial aspect of the wrist, depending on the plane of transfer. It should be placed so that the turning back of the trap-door leaves the raw area in one plane. In this way, the trap-door lies smoothly back when suturing is complete and the attachment as a whole runs cleanly off the limb.

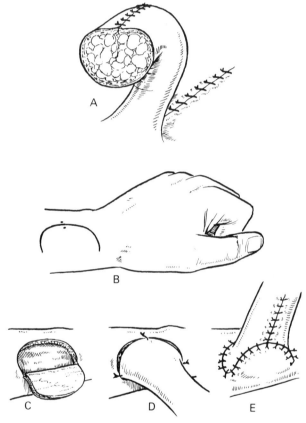

Fig. 4.15 Transfer of a flap by wrist carrier. With the single pedicled flap raised as in Figure 4.14 a circular raw surface is left when tubing has been completed (A) and a semicircular trapdoor (B) is outlined and raised (C) to give a circular raw surface to correspond to (A) and the two are sutured together (D and E).

The other variable is the angle of attachment and consideration of how arm and wrist are going to lie at the next transfer and the angle which arm and pedicle must make as a result should decide this. The 'hinge' along which the trap-door is raised will be perpendicular to the desired direction of the flap.

Before detaching the flap and before raising a single pedicle flap, it is wise to tattoo suitable points, e.g. centre and margins of the pedicle, so that fixing sutures to distribute suture-line tension can be used. The difficult healing point is where the trap-door meets the axial scar of the tubed pedicle and care in suturing here is advisable.

Waltzing (Fig. 4.16). The primary defect, that is the defect which the flap was designed to reconstruct, is being filled in greater part by the transferred distal segment. It is only in the rare event of a multistaged waltzed transfer with movement of each end of the flap

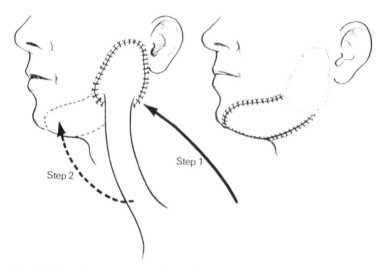

Fig. 4.16 Transfer of a flap by waltzing. Part of the primary defect is covered with Step 1 of the transfer and the remainder at Step 2. *Between completion of Step 1 and the carrying out of Step 2 a delay as shown in Figure 4.17 is essential.*

in turn that the matter of siting a trap-door arises. The steps then differ from those described for the carrier method only in the siting of the trap-door with a view to achieving the maximum of movement in the desired direction commensurate with the minimum of kinking and tension during both the current and the subsequent transfer.

The use of delay

Delay as used to allow a random pattern flap to have a more advantageous length-breadth ratio or allow increase in length of an axial pattern flap beyond its recognised safe dimensions has already been discussed on p. 111.

The same basic manoeuvre may also be needed at other stages of flap transfer, particularly in the case of an axial pattern flap (Fig. 4.17). When such a flap has been attached to a wrist carrier or has been inset in the process of a waltzing transfer the next stage of the transfer involves division of the base of the flap, i.e. its pedicle. This has the effect of cutting off its axial vascular flow and the flap is immediately downgraded to the status of a random pattern flap, the equivalent of a tube pedicle. Division of the pedicle in this way also means that the flap is required forthwith to survive on the vascular throughflow it has established via its carrier or waltzing inset. This may not be adequate to ensure its survival. The efficiency of its pre-existing arteriovenous axis is such that there is obviously little encouragement for the flap to develop an effective new vascular attachment at the inset. The efficiency of the new vascular attachment requires to be enhanced before it is likely to be capable of sustaining the entire flap and this is achieved by a staged reduction in the efficiency of the pedicle which contains the arteriovenous axis.

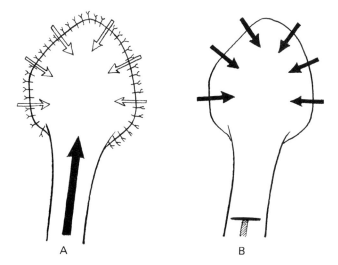

Fig. 4.17 The use of a delay to enhance the flow of blood across the distal attachment of an axial pattern flap. In A, the contrast between the vigorous axial vascular flow and the poor blood flow across the distal attachment prior to delay is contrasted with the situation (B) following delay with division of the axial vasculature and resulting enhancement of the blood flow across the distal attachment.

In practice a 'delay' of the pedicle is carried out with partial division, usually one third to one half of its cross-sectional area, but, more important, with division of the axial vessels. The effect is to alter the vascular dynamics of the flap and improve the efficiency of perfusion through the wrist or waltzing inset.

Such a delay is usually carried out three weeks after the initial transfer to wrist or waltzing inset and it is essential that in carrying it out the axial vessels, most of all the axial artery, should be formally demonstrated, ligated and divided. Full division of the pedicle is carried out a week later.

Failure to stage division in this way is liable to result in substantial flap necrosis. Staging of the division even of a random pattern flap such as a tube pedicle is also sometimes advisable if the blood flow across an attachment is regarded as doubtfully adequate.

Flap division and insetting

When the flap applied to a defect is having its pedicle divided prior to return of its bridge segment to its donor site and completion of insetting it is sometimes advisable to separate division and insetting into distinct stages (Fig. 4.18). Completion of insetting involves dissecting the flap back off the original inset for a varying distance to allow it to sit neatly. This has an adverse effect on the blood supply of the segment which has been elevated and its margin may slough producing the phenomenon of 'rim' necrosis.

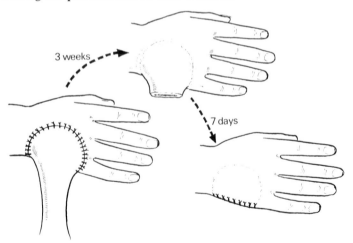

Fig. 4.18 Staged division of a tubed flap and insetting. The pedicle of the flap is divided at the end of the third week, but insetting is postponed for a further week in order to avoid rim necrosis. The method as used in direct flap transfer is shown in Figure 4.39.

Outside the head and neck it is wise routinely to postpone insetting the flap for a week after division of its pedicle. It is safe more often to divide and inset immediately in the head and neck because of the rich blood supply of the whole area but even there the least doubt should mean a staged division and inset.

Assessment of circulatory adequacy

It is generally accepted that an inset flap takes about three weeks to develop across the inset a vascular flow capable of perfusing the flap entirely on its own. In the hope of reducing this time several tests have been introduced and each in turn discarded, each aiming to assess the efficiency of the vascular attachment under consideration. Most of these tests have involved measuring the passage of substances such as atropine, fluorescein and $Na^{24}CL$ across the inset and using this to assess efficiency. Fluorescein is at present enjoying a second honeymoon.

The problem really is that these tests are measuring quite indirectly and rather dubiously those factors which need to be measured, namely the *vis a tergo* of the blood entering the pedicle and the overall adequacy of the venous drainage.

In any case flaps fail to complete their transfer within the recognised time scale because of necrosis more often than for any other reason. To risk necrosis in an attempt to save a few days shows a lack of maturity on the part of the clinician.

The question more often should be whether the transfer is safe even at three weeks and in such an assessment additional evidence such as adequacy of deep, as well as marginal attachment, speed of healing, presence of induration and reaction locally are all factors used in conjunction with local vascular reactions in decision taking.

THE PLANNING OF FLAPS

Defining the defect

Before repair by a flap is contemplated the extent of the defect must be defined in terms of each component—skin, bone and lining. In this the quality of the skin surrounding the obvious defect must be taken into account. Skin showing radiotherapy damage or the fibrotic and atrophic changes of old scarring is not good surgical material and is often better regarded as part of the defect and excised in order to reach the good skin beyond it (Fig. 4.19). In addition to its poor suture-holding qualities the avascularity of such skin makes it unsatisfactory for nourishing a pedicle inset when the remainder of the pedicle is detached for transfer. A good criterion, skin texture and appearance apart, is the state of skin mobility; skin freely mobile deeply is usually reasonably satisfactory to work with.

Planning the procedure

Planning has two distinct parts which, while they cannot be quite

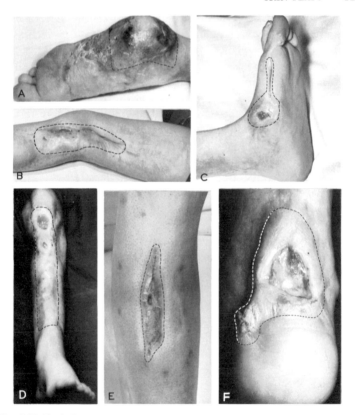

Fig. 4.19 Typical areas suitable for flap cover and the extent of excision required solely to eliminate scarring. It should be appreciated that further skin may have to be excised to permit the flap to have a shape suitable from a vascular viewpoint. Thus Figure 4.42B shows the flap used to repair the defect F. Stages in the repair of A are shown in Figures 4.8D, 4.20 and 4.42D, and of D in Figures 4.43C and 4.44B.

divorced in practice, are best considered separately. They consist of **deciding the type of flap** and **planning the actual transfer**.

Type of flap
The transfer of a flap may involve moving tissue **adjoining the defect**, i.e. local flap, or tissue **at a distance** from it.

Local flap. Before local tissue can be transferred it must be demonstrably available and ways of assessing the size of the local flap required for a particular defect will be described under the heading Rotation and Transposed Flaps (see p. 133).

Distant flap. The transfer of tissue from a distance follows one of three patterns:

1. The defect is brought to the flap. This type of transfer has its

main use in defects of the forearm and hands. If the defect can be brought within the reach of an axial pattern flap source, such a flap should be the first choice. The less satisfactory alternative is a random pattern flap raised on the trunk and applied to the defect. In this context both flaps are regarded as direct flaps.

2. The defect and the flap are each brought to the other. Both the donor area and the defect are moved into close proximity to each other so that a flap can be transferred directly from one to the other. This is the situation when a direct flap is transferred from leg to leg—a cross-leg flap; from forearm to opposite hand—a cross-arm flap; or from finger to finger—a cross-finger flap.

3. The flap is brought to the defect. In this transfer the defect remains virtually static and the bulk of the movement involved in the transfer is done by the flap. The movement may take the form of waltzing the flap to the defect if the two are reasonably near one another or by using a wrist carrier when the two are further apart.

The appropriate type of flap in any set instance tends to be governed by the **size** and **site** of the defect and the **time factor** in the transfer.

Size of the defect. A local flap has to be much greater in area than the defect it is planned to cover and the limbs are seldom able to provide enough tissue to cover the size of limb defect which commonly requires flap cover. In the trunk and face the necessary area of tissue is more likely to be present and the local flap is more often a practical possibility.

The area of tissue which is readily transferred as a direct flap is smaller than that transferred on a wrist carrier, and large defects usually require a distant flap, carried on the wrist or waltzed to the defect.

Site of the defect. A direct flap can only be used if the defect and donor area can be brought into proximity readily and this limits its usage to defects of arm and hand, lower leg and foot. In other sites a distant flap has to be used, waltzed or using a carrier.

The time factor. The local flap is often virtually completed in a single stage and may be desirable on this score. It does not involve the patient in maintaining a particular position for a period of time with consequent liability to joint stiffness (see p. 159) as do both the direct flap and tube pedicle. The need to maintain a position for a prolonged period with the bed rest which this may entail can be a contra-indication in the older age group to the use of a direct flap or other distant flap.

The transfer of a direct flap is completed in 4 to 5 weeks, an axial pattern flap waltzed to its destination takes about the same time, carried on the wrist takes about 7 weeks, while a classic tube pedicle takes 12 weeks and often longer.

The direct flap and the axial pattern flap waltzed can be used as an emergency procedure; the tube pedicle and the axial pattern flap carried on the wrist can only be used in an elective manner beciause of the need for prior stages in the transfer.

A further factor which may influence the selection of the type of flap, in particular whether it should be local or distant, is the characteristics, cosmetic and otherwise, of the transferred tissue.

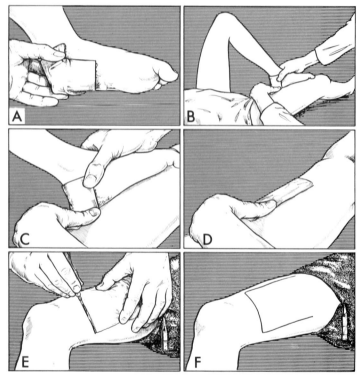

Fig. 4.20 Planning in reverse. The area (Fig. 4.19A) requiring replacement is covered with the jaconet 'flap' (A), the legs are placed in the transfer position and (B and C) the 'flap' is put into the position it will take during the actual transfer (*see* Fig. 4.42D). The 'flap' is then laid out on the donor area (D) and outlined with Bonney's Blue (E) to give the shape and position of the actual flap (F).

After transfer, flap skin retains very much the appearance and other characteristics which it had prior to transfer. Transferred to a mobile part of the face, abdominal or chest skin tends to be mask-like because the fine play of facial movements cannot be transmitted through the thicker trunk skin, even when it has been completely defatted. Transferred to the heel, abdominal skin lacks the characteristics of the local skin (quite apart from its sensory perception) which enable it to weight-bear successfully.

Planning the transfer

With the type of flap decided, its site, size and shape, and the stages of the transfer are planned by the method of *planning in reverse* (Fig. 4.20). The defect is outlined with a suitable material such as jaconet. With this representing the flap the procedure is carried from the end result backwards through the various stages with the limbs in their correct position until the 'flap' ends up on the skin area from which it is to be taken, where it is used to outline the definitive flap. In this way the patient is not given an impossible position to maintain at a critical stage of the transfer and the surgeon avoids a flap which is too small, one which will kink during transfer or fail to reach its destination because it is too short. Time spent on the planning stage is never wasted in the long run.

A flap should always be planned with a margin of reserve.

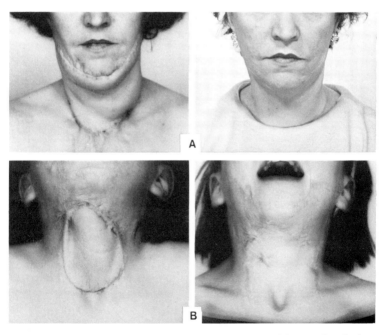

Fig. 4.21 The result immediately following the completion of the transfer of tube pedicles to correct postburn neck contractures and after Z-plasties coupled with thinning. A previous stage in the transfer of A is shown in Figure 4.44B and the tube pedicle used for B is shown in Figure 4.43D.

Skimping, making it just neat, will certainly create difficulties for the surgeon in due course. It is easy to trim an excessively large flap, but difficult to add to one, once begun.

The exigencies of blood supply may dictate dimensions, shape and thickness which would not be necessary otherwise, and subsequent trimming, thinning and Z-plasties have often to be carried out after the flap has completed its transfer to give the optimal result (Fig. 4.21).

ROTATION AND TRANSPOSED FLAPS

To cover a primary defect it may be possible to move the adjoining tissue, any secondary defect being closed by direct suture or free skin graft. When the tissue is rotated into the primary defect the flap is called a **rotation flap**; moved laterally into the defect it is called a **transposed flap**. Most flaps combine both principles in varying degrees and a particular flap may be called by the principle which predominates (Fig. 4.22).

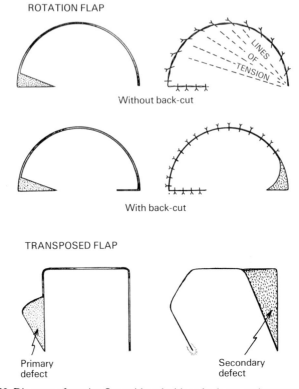

Fig. 4.22 Diagrams of rotation flaps with and without back-cut, and transposed flap.

These flaps cannot adequately be described in print, even with a profusion of illustrative examples (Figs. 4.23, 4.24, 4.25 and 4.26), for every flap is an individual problem. In the face particularly,

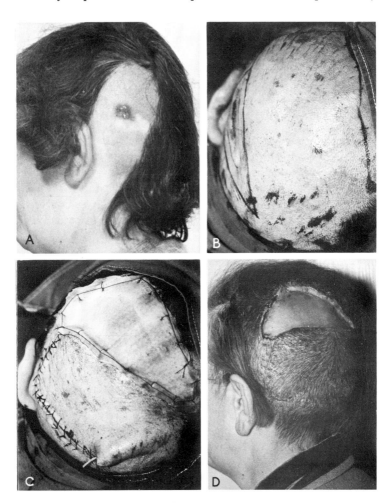

Fig. 4.23 Transposed flap used following excision of rodent ulcer involving outer table of skull. Flap outlined after triangulation of defect to be left when the ulcer (A) is widely excised (B). The flap transferred (C) and the secondary defect covered with a split-skin graft. The final result (D).

judgment in selection and imagination in design come with the experience born in surgical apprenticeship. Present discussion is concerned to explain the principles underlying the construction of such flaps. They depend to a considerable extent on the elasticity of the tissues, but in planning this should not be relied on; rather it should be considered as an added insurance. They are geometrical manoeuvres and treated as such are more likely to be trouble-free in practice.

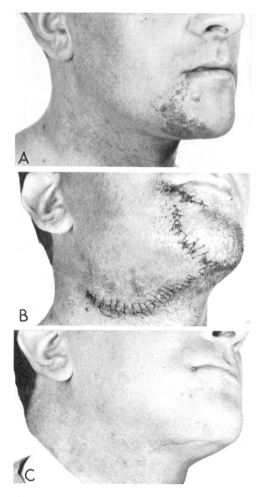

Fig. 4.24 Rotation flap without back-cut following excision of haemangioma.

It must be stressed before describing these local flaps in detail that they are not procedures to be lightly embarked upon. The surgeon using such a flap should remember always that a major vascular disaster is liable to leave a deformity far greater than the one the flap was designed to relieve.

Principle of rotation (Fig. 4.27)
As the flap will be rotated into position it should in theory be the arc

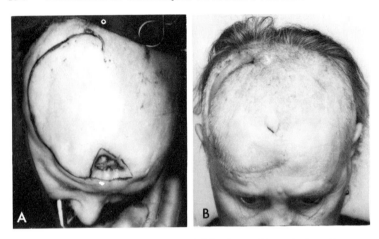

Fig. 4.25 Rotation flap with back-cut used following excision of rodent ulcer involving outer table of skull. Flap outlined (A) after triangulating the defect to be left after excision of the ulcer. Final result (B) with the secondary defect split-skin grafted.

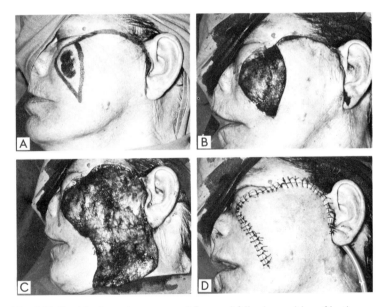

Fig. 4.26 Combined rotation-transposed flap used following excision of lentigo maligna of cheek. Flap outlined (A), raised (B, C), and transferred (D).

of a circle of which the primary defect is a segment, flap and defect together making a half-circle. The defect is thus approximately triangular in shape and the narrower the triangle the less does the tissue have to rotate to fill the defect. With the flap rotated into the

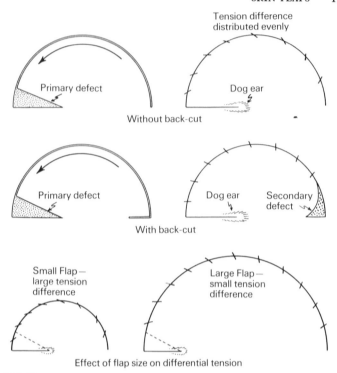

Fig. 4.27 Diagrams of rotation flaps showing the effect of the back-cut and the influence of the size of the flap on tension difference.

defect and sutured in place there is a difference of tension on the two sides of the suture line and ideally this difference of tension is distributed evenly all along the suture line. It follows that the larger the circle of the flap, the longer is the line along which the tension difference can be distributed and the smaller the difference at any particular point. The rotation flap usually relies so much for its success on the laxity of the tissues that it is really impossible to give an accurate site for the point around which the flap pivots.

A **pure** rotation flap has no secondary defect but often, depending on the laxity of the tissues and the degree of rotation required, the primary defect cannot be closed purely by redistributing the tension and a further incision has to be made to allow the flap to move laterally as well as rotate into the defect. Where the curve of flap and defect makes a half circle the incision is made as a back-cut along the diameter line. This enables the flap to move by a combination of rotation and transposition into the defect.

This back-cut creates a secondary defect which is closed where possible by direct suture, failing this by a free skin graft.

Principle of transposition

Even in its purest form the transposed flap does pivot on an axis and so does rotate, but the major movement is lateral. The primary defect is again triangular and the rectangular flap constructed along one of its sides moves laterally when transposed into the defect. One purpose of the manoeuvre is to avoid tension of the suture line closing the primary defect and so the secondary defect cannot be directly sutured since this would recreate the very tension the flap was designed to avoid. It must therefore be closed either by a free skin graft or by a further plastic procedure which will permit closure without tension.

The vascular limitations of local flaps

When a local flap is moved there tends to be a line of tension along the base or obliquely across the flap and this, if excessive, is prone to cause necrosis of the tissue beyond it. A back-cut will usually eliminate the tension line and allow the flap to move readily into the defect, but it must be recognised that the back-cut also reduces the vascular area of the base and thus the circulatory reserve.

These two factors—vascular area and tension—must always be balanced and to know just how much one may be reduced to eliminate the other in a particular situation is a measure of experience. Probably tension is a more potent producer of massive necrosis than reduction of vascular area. The enhancement of vascular efficiency produced by a delay tends to be offset by the fibrosis which it causes particularly if the delay includes elevation of the flap for the flexibility of a flap always helps to reduce tension.

Planning the flap (Fig. 4.28)

It must be stated at the outset that the guiding principles to be laid down apply to rotation and transposed flaps in their classical forms and do not necessarily apply to many of the flaps used in certain parts of the head and neck. These will be discussed separately.

The first step with either type of flap is to **triangulate the defect**. The defect must be capable of being outlined as a triangle with two sides approximately equal and this may necessitate the sacrifice of normal tissue to make the triangle. A defect which for any reason cannot be triangulated is seldom suitable for a standard local flap. As a rule the two equal sides of the triangle are longer than the third which forms the base and in visualising the procedure and the flap appropriate to it the defect must be thought of as being closed by moving one of the equal sides as a side of the flap across to the other.

With a long, narrow defect, triangulation may be planned to place

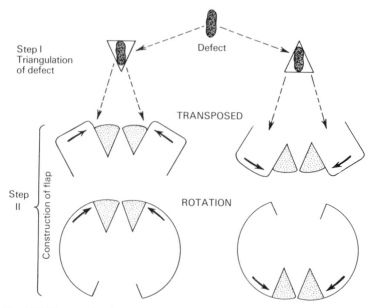

Step I
Triangulation
of defect

Defect

TRANSPOSED

ROTATION

Step II

Construction of flap

Fig. 4.28 The steps in planning a local flap.
Step I selects the direction of the base of the flap—transposed or rotation.
Step II selects the side of the defect from which the flap is to be moved.

the apex at either end, and which end should be apex and which base may not be immediately apparent. The base of the flap will be alongside the apex of the triangle and so the end should be chosen as apex which will provide the better flap base from the point of view of blood supply, line of scar and tissue availability.

With the triangle defined, it may at once be obvious from which side the flap will come. If there is doubt, two factors will decide:

1. The side with most tissue available is likely to provide the best flap.

2. The anatomical distribution of blood vessels may clearly favour one side.

The flap must next be outlined and the principles of construction depend on whether it is to be transposed or rotated.

The transposed flap (Fig. 4.29)
The ideal length-breadth ratio varies with the site, but the flap should be approximately square and in a difficult situation its demensions should be even more favourable. Only in the head and neck is a flap which is longer than it is broad safe and even there the nearer the flap is to a square the safer it is.

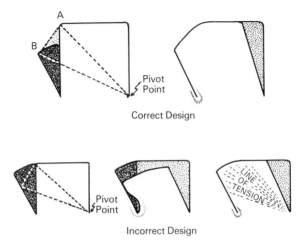

Correct Design

Incorrect Design

Fig. 4.29 The design of a transposed flap. Compare the well-designed flap where the distance from the pivot point to A equals that to B and the transfer is consequently without tension, and the incorrectly designed flap where the distances are unequal because the flap is too short and the transfer can only be achieved with tension.

The classical shape then is square, and in planning it must first be recognised that the point around which the flap will pivot in moving is not the apex of the triangle, but rather the other side of the base of the flap. From this it follows that if the flap is to close the defect the distance from the pivotal point to the far point of the triangle must equal the diagonal length of the flap from the pivotal point.

Before any incision is made the pivot point must be clearly defined and the distance from the pivot to each point of the flap compared with its estimated distance to the same point when transposition is complete. Where the distance before transposition is shorter there will be a line of tension along that line when the flap is transposed. The diagonal length of the flap from the pivot point in the square flap is the one particularly liable to be short. The distances can be equated in two ways:

1. *Initial design.* The flap can be made longer than the side of the triangulated defect so that its actual diagonal length before and estimated diagonal length after transfer are equal and the shape and dimensions of the flap can be similarly decided by considering actual lengths before and estimated lengths after.

This is the best method and the one to be used in planning the flap. If, however, it should be found when the flap has been cut that the length is inadequate and a tension line will result, an alternative but on the whole less satisfactory device must be used, namely the back-cut. *Indeed to have to use a back-cut is an admission of bad initial design.*

2. *The back-cut.* As the flap has been cut in length is fixed and so the point of pivot must be altered to reduce the discrepancies of length. A back-cut achieves this. Though it does reduce tension it must be remembered that it also reduces vascularity and so should be as small as possible. Sometimes it proves possible to reduce the tension without significantly reducing the vascularity by cutting only the actual tissue responsible for the tension leaving at the same time the blood vessels intact. In skin with a good thickness of superficial fascia section of the skin alone may give enough relaxation, while in the scalp cutting the galea aponeurotica may have the same result. In the face and neck such differential section is seldom feasible, but fortunately blood supply and tissue availability are usually so good that the problem is less likely to arise in an acute form.

The transposed flap is especially useful where a secondary graft is not contra-indicated for cosmetic reasons and so it is used mainly outside the face. With it the size of the secondary defect approximates in area to the primary defect and it is covered with a split-skin graft. Any attempt to close the secondary defect by direct suture destroys the whole point of the flap transfer for the reason already given. The graft can be applied either primarily, using pressure methods, or delayed, using exposed grafting. Delayed grafting has the virtue of ensuring that any haematoma collecting under the flap can freely drain into the secondary defect and not add to any tension in the flap itself. If it is decided to graft the secondary defect primarily it is essential to make sure that the tension on the bolus tie-over dressing is not transmitted to the flap. This can be ensured quite simply by anchoring both the flap margin and the graft to the deeper tissues. Making sure that the tie-over sutures passing through the margin of the flap include the deep tissues in their bite has this effect. Suturing in this way also allows the flap to be managed quite independently of the graft from the point of view of suction, pressure dressings, etc. (Fig. 4.30).

The rotation flap (Fig. 4.31)

The classical rotation flap has a near circular curve and, used with or without a back-cut along the diameter of the semicircle, the curve of the flap is able to rotate along the corresponding curve of the other side of the incision outlining the flap. It is sutured in its new position with a degree of differential tension, but when a back-cut is needed in addition, as it frequently is, a triangular secondary defect is

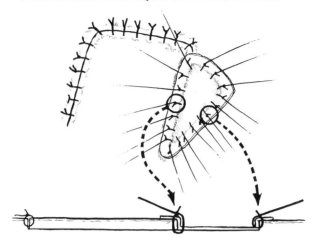

Fig. 4.30 Isolation of flap from the graft by use of sutures anchoring graft and flap to the deeper structures. This manoeuvre prevents tension being transmitted between graft and flap and allows them to be handled independently of one another.

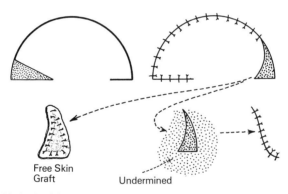

Free Skin Graft

Undermined

Fig. 4.31 Methods of closing the secondary defect following transfer of a rotation flap by free skin grafting and direct suture.

opened up and the flap really then combines rotation and transposition. With the movement of curve on curve there is no defect in the region of the actual flap except at the back-cut. The larger the flap is made the less the difference of tension at each point of the flap and most difficulties arise from planning on too small rather than on too large a scale.

The point around which the flap pivots lies approximately midway between the apex of the triangular defect and the end of the back-cut, and the distance from this point to each point of the flap must equal its distance to the point to which it will be sutured after rotation. The pivot of the rotation flap cannot be pinpointed with the accuracy possible in the transposed flap for the rotation flap does rely to a considerable extent on the flexibility of the tissues. It is because of this that it generally works best when the skin is lax and flexible.

Outside the head and neck the secondary defect is routinely split-skin grafted and in actual practice suturing of the flap is stopped as soon as tension is clearly present and the graft is applied. In the head and neck the secondary defect is usually closed by direct suture with the proviso that such closure must not create tension along the base of the flap sufficient to jeopardise its blood supply. If direct closure is impossible a graft must be used.

The problem of the secondary defect left when the flap is rotated can sometimes be solved in quite a different way (Fig. 4.32) which is best understood by considering the relative wound lengths. The length of the flap is less than that of the wound to which it has to be sutured and the two lengths can be equated either by increasing the length of the flap side, which is the effect of the back-cut, or by reducing the length of the outer line of the wound to make it equal the length of the flap. Excising a triangle of tissue opposite where the back-cut would normally be has just this effect and is feasible when there is enough tissue available to allow excision. In the event the flap is rotated without back-cut and as suturing proceeds it becomes obvious that there is some redundant tissue on the outer side of the suture line and eventually a dog-ear develops, excision of which leaves the two sides equal in length. It is only in the head and neck that there is spare tissue available to allow this method to be used.

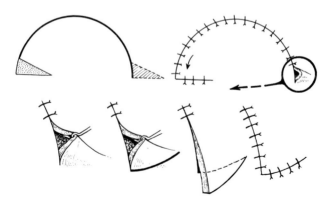

Fig. 4.32 A method of avoiding a secondary defect which can sometimes be used when the skin is lax and tissue available in consequence. Figure 6.19 shows the method in practice.

The dog-ear of the triangulated defect

If the pivoting took place round the apex of the triangulated primary defect the resulting suture line would be quite flat but with the pivot point elsewhere both in the rotated and transposed flap there tends to be a dog-ear left at the apex of the triangle when the flap is moved. Though it may be possible to deal with this in the usual way at the time of flap transfer, it should always be left for subsequent excision if its removal would in any way jeopardise the blood supply of the flap.

FLAPS OF HEAD AND NECK

Although classical local flaps are often used in the head and neck the extremely rich vascular pattern coupled with a laxity of tissue greater than elsewhere in the body permit the planning and execution of flaps with less regard for the usual requirements than would be necessary elsewhere. Most of these flaps are random in type, but in

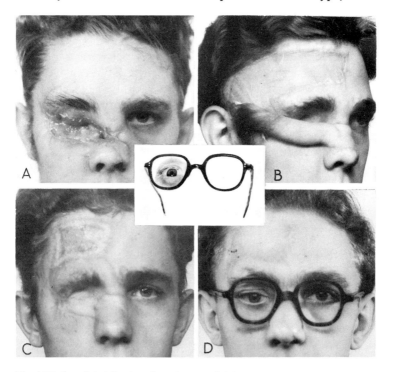

Fig. 4.33 A pedicled flap based on the superficial temporal vascular pattern. The post-traumatic scarring with loss of eyeball and severe damage to eyelids (A) is replaced by the flap (B), the forehead defect being split-skin grafted. With the carrier segment returned to its original site the final result is shown without (C), and with (D), the prosthesis (inset).

addition a commonly used flap in the head and neck is the axial type—long and narrow, based on a known arteriovenous system.

Examples are the temporal flap based on the superficial temporal vessels (Fig. 4.33), and the Indian forehead flap based on the supraorbital vessels (Fig. 4.34).

In most of these the greater part of the flap is used as a carrier of the terminal segment which alone is set into the defect. Three weeks suffice for the inset segment to establish its vascular supply locally; the flap is divided and the unused carrier segment is returned whence it came. It is fortunate that the copious vascular pattern permits the carrier segment to be left raw on its deep surface without fear of disastrous sepsis for the narrowness of these flaps relative to their bulk would make tubing impossible.

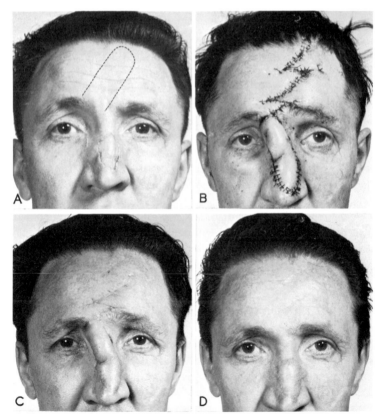

Fig. 4.34 A forehead flap based on the supra-orbital vascular pattern. The scarring (A), the end result of a very extensive kerato-acanthoma, is replaced by the flap (B and C), the forehead defect being closed by direct suture incorporating Z-plasties. Final result (D).

Where the defect left by raising the flap cannot be closed by direct suture a split-skin graft is used for temporary cover and this is removed in due course when the carrier segment is returned to its original site. The graft convering the donor site of the transferred segment is usually left as a permanency.

Flap planning

With a piece of jaconet shaped to represent the proposed flap and its pedicle held in correct position, the 'flap' is transferred to make sure that it is capable of reaching its destination and the jaconet shape is then used to outline the definitive flap. Time and care spent on this step will prevent the disaster of the flap which only reaches its destination with difficulty or not at all.

Flap transfer

The precise thinness of tissue required in the defect can often be duplicated in the flap with safety, so abundant is the blood supply, but in passing from the part of the flap to be inset to the carrier segment the flap should be broadened and thickened to allow for maximal blood supply. For the purposes of flap thickness the head can be divided into the vault of the skull as far as the margins of the galea aponeurotica where the blood supply is entirely marginal and the routine plane of dissection is the loose areolar tissue deep to the galea, and the remaining skin which of course has an additional deep blood supply. As a result delay of a scalp flap need never include elevation.

In the forehead the terminal flap may safely be made thin enough to leave the frontalis muscle behind and in the face and neck it may include the minimum of fat, but in both instances it should thicken fairly rapidly to the more usual plane of dissection. In the neck this plane is best deep to platysma and includes as much of the superficial venous system as possible.

Returning the carrier segment

During the three weeks the carrier segment tends to tube itself in two distinct ways, by fibrotic contraction of the raw surface and by marginal epithelialisation. When returning it to its original site, the fibrous tissue must be excised completely to undo the tubing and to get the best suture line the marginal epithelium should also be removed. Even so, the flap tends to remain a trifle narrower than when it was originally raised and when suturing it back in position after removing the temporary graft the scalp may have to be mobilised quite widely to bring the skin edges readily together. This is most likely to occur if the graft has been applied with the scalp in the naturally retracted position it assumes when the flap is raised. It is possible to overcome retraction of the scalp by suturing the temporary graft under slightly greater than normal tension. This reduction of the grafted area to a minimum makes the subsequent replacement of the flap much more straightforward and free of tension.

Following division and return of the carrier segment the insetting of the transferred segment of the flap is completed and as in the direct flap a little thinning of the margin may be necessary to allow it to sit neatly into the defect.

Flaps based either on the superficial temporal or supra-orbital vessels tend to be the most useful in the repair of sizeable defects of the face above the level of the mouth—generally of the nose, cheek and lower eyelid.

The first point to be considered in planning is whether the skin cover is to be hairy or not for this will decide whether scalp or forehead must provide the skin. Thereafter the appropriate pedicle can be selected using jaconet to give the exact outline. A supra-orbital based flap works well for symmetrical nasal defects; defects of one side can be covered with either type—supra-orbital or temporal. When the defect involves cheek, either alone or with part of the nose, the temporal flap is usually more satisfactory as the length of pedicle gives the flap a longer reach.

While it is often necessary to provide lining as well as skin cover the methods used to provide such lining are beyond the scope of this book and will not be discussed further.

Flaps are often required to repair the defects which follow excision of neoplastic lesions, simple, premalignant and malignant, which are unsuited for repair by direct suture or free skin graft. They may also be used to replace a free skin graft used for primary repair which is unsatisfactory cosmetically. This subject will be discussed in more detail in chapter 6.

In acute trauma, as described in chapter 1, flaps have a very limited use and should be attempted only by an experienced plastic surgeon.

AXIAL PATTERN FLAPS OF TRUNK

The axial pattern flaps which have become established are the **deltopectoral**, the **groin** and the **hypogastric** flaps.

The deltopectoral flap (Fig. 4.35)

The deltopectoral flap has as its axial vascular basis the perforating branches of the internal mammary vessels. It lies transversely on the anterior chest wall with its base medial, along the border of the sternum. The usual upper border is the line of the clavicle, the lower is the anterior axiallary fold. The lateral extent of the vascular

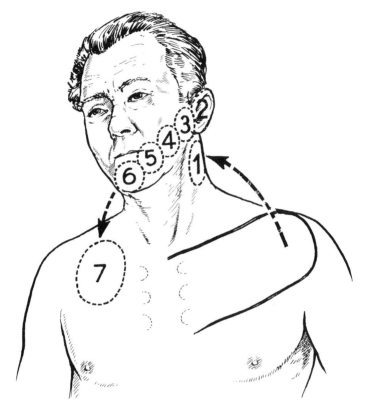

Fig. 4.35 The common sites on the head, neck and chest, suitable for cover with the deltopectoral flap.

territory of the perforating vessels is not uniform but clinical experience has shown that the deltopectoral flap, raised deep to the fascia, stripping the underlying muscle bare, can safely extend on to the anterior surface of the deltoid muscle. A flap raised within these lines and conforming to their general configuration can safely be raised without prior delay. If length greater than this is required, a preliminary delay of the segment distal to the line separating deltoid from pectoralis major is wise. The only artery of size divided in raising the flap is often the deltoid branch of the acromiothoracic axis and if a delay is being carried out this vessel should be sought and formally divided. The flap can safely be raised almost to the sternal margin, where the axial vessels emerge into it, one in each intercostal space. The second perforating vessel, judged on comparative size, is the most important of the three or four usually incorporated in the flap.

The bridge segment is usually tubed; if suction is being used the catheter can be inserted along the length of the tube.

The secondary defect is split-skin grafted and the site is an ideal one for delayed exposed grafting. The defect is an extensive one and, grafted in its entirety, leaves a considerable area of grafted skin to be excised when the bridge segment is returned to its pre-operative site following division of the pedicle three weeks after the initial transfer. In the light of this there is much to be said for grafting only the area finally left on the deltoid as the permanent secondary defect. The remainder can be treated as a temporary raw surface and merely dressed (Fig. 4.36).

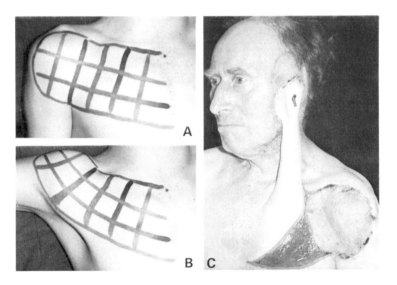

Fig. 4.36 Demonstration of the slack skin available along the anterior axillary fold (A and B) with (C) an example of deltopectoral flap used to resurface a defect left following amputation of the ear for squamous carcinoma.

Used to resurface defects in its vicinity, the deltopectoral flap is most often moved upwards, the lower face and neck being a more prolific source of defects than the lower chest. In this role it can readily be moved in a quarter circle (Fig. 4.35) to cover defects anywhere within its arc—mastoid region, ear, parotid, cheek, mouth and chin—waltzed on its sternal attachment. It is capable of reaching about as high as the zygomatic arch, a range which can of course be extended by preliminary delay on to the end of the standard flap. The zygomatic arch is actually higher than planning measurements would appear to permit, taking the pivot point to be the medial end of the lower border of the flap. This anomaly is explained by the fact that the lower border lies along the anterior axillary fold where there is a large amount of slack skin available, taken up when the arm is abducted. The inequality in length between the two borders of the flap which this slack creates means that any tension line developed during transfer tends to be along the shorter upper border and not the longer lower border. In planning, therefore, the effective length of the flap should be measured along the upper border with the pivot point at its medial end (Fig. 4.36).

Though the most common transfer of the deltopectoral flap is upwards it can be rotated to any area on the chest and upper abdomen within its reach and is, in addition, used to resurface the hand, palm or dorsum (p. 256).

The groin flap (Fig. 8.12)

The groin flap uses as its arteriovenous axial system the superficial circumflex iliac (Fig. 4.37). It is based medially and lies along the line of the groin. Relying as it does on a single artery the anatomy of this vessel is of importance to ensure that it is invariably incorporated in the flap. The artery arises 2–3 cm below the inguinal ligament, usually from the femoral artery, occasionally from the superficial epigastric artery at its origin. It runs laterally, parallel to the inguinal ligament, and at the medial border of sartorius gives a deep branch. From that point it becomes more superficial passing into the tissue which would be raised as a groin flap. Lateral to the anterior superior iliac spine it divides and is no longer regularly identifiable. The corresponding vein has a general pattern parallel to the artery ending at the saphenous opening which is very close to the origin of the artery.

In planning the flap the anterior superior iliac spine, the pubic tubercle and the intervening inguinal ligament are marked on the skin. The line of the femoral artery can be palpated and on it 2.5 cm below the inguinal ligment the origin of the superficial circumflex iliac artery is marked. The line of the vessel is then drawn parallel to the inguinal ligament and its point of entry into the flap can be marked where the vessel crosses the medial border of sartorius. With these skin markings the flap can be planned to include the artery

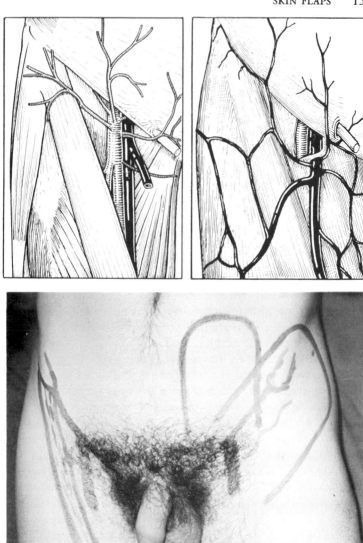

Fig. 4.37 The vascular anatomy of the inguinal region (arterial, modified from Gray, venous, after Testut) which provides the axial arteriovenous basis of the groin and hypogastric flaps, and the skin markings used in raising the flaps in practice.

though it need not necessarily lie along the central axis of the flap. Usual width is 10 cm but extremes of 6 cm and 19 cm in an adult and 14 cm in a child have been used quite successfully. The safe maximum length is difficult to define since the lateral extent of the vascular territory is not known with certainty, but if the flap is raised beyond the anterior superior iliac spine, the part of the flap beyond this should be square, i.e. with a 1:1 length to breadth ratio.

The flap should be raised at the level of the deep fascia. In making the upper marginal incision it is usual to divide the superficial epigastric vessels and if the flap is raised through a plane deep to this it is certain to include its axial vessels since the two sets of vessels, superficial epigastric and superficial circumflex iliac are on the same plane. The key point in raising the flap is the virtually constant branching of the artery at the medial border of sartorius. When sartorius is reached the fascia overlying it should be incised and the muscle stripped bare to just short of its medial border. Dissection can usually stop there in the knowledge that the artery is safely out of the way.

The width of the secondary defect can be reduced by flexing the hip, a manoeuvre which allows most to be closed by direct suture. If grafting is unavoidable the method to be used depends on whether or not the secondary defect is overlaid by the flap. If it is overlaid primary grafting with a tie-over dressing is unavoidable; if it is not overlaid delayed exposed grafting is a possible alternative whose use reduces the magnitude of the procedure.

The groin flap can be used in one of three ways—to resurface the hand, as a local flap and as a tube pedicle. In this last role it can be raised and immediately attached to the wrist as a carrier on its radial or ulnar side as in Figure 4.15 saving the six-week period of maturation required for the classic tube pedicle.

The hypogastric flap (Fig. 4.38)
This flap uses as its arteriovenous axial system the superficial epigastric (Fig. 4.37). It is an inferiorly based flap raised on the lower abdomen with its axis passing upwards and slightly laterally from the line of the inguinal ligament at approximately its midpoint. The flap has been designed varying in length from 5–18 cm and in width from 3–7 cm. It is raised at the level of Scarpa's fascia as two parallel incisions tapering to a point above, as far down as the inguinal ligament. It has been used mainly for resurfacing the hand, though it would equally be available as a local flap.

The management of the secondary defect parallels that of the groin flap.

Subsequent stages of transfer. With all three flaps the next stage of transfer is carried out three weeks after raising the flap.

When the defect for which the flap is being used has been virtually covered by the flap its management parallels that of a direct flap.

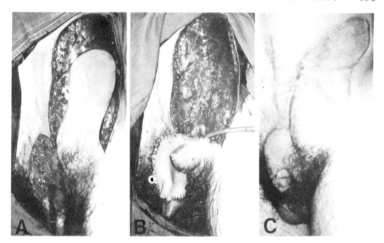

Fig. 4.38 The hypogastric flap, used as a local flap to replace suprapubic scarring, part of an epispadias. The use of suction catheter drainage under the flap is also shown in B.
A The hypogastric flap cut, ready for transfer to the suprapubic defect.
B The flap transferred and sutured in position.
C The end result with the secondary defect split-skin grafted and the bridge segment of the flap returned to its original site.

The bridge segment is divided completely but insetting is postponed for a further week to avoid rim necrosis.

As with all axial pattern flaps, and for the reasons given on p. 126, when a significant proportion of the flap remains to be inset, or when the flap is being used as a tube pedicle, a delay is carried out at the end of the third week with ligation and division of the axial artery a formal step in the procedure. With the axial vessel cut off in this way the flap of course ceases to have any significant characteristics which distinguish it from a random pattern flap and in any subsequent management it is handled as one.

THE DIRECT FLAP

The direct flap generally has a random pattern of blood vessels. It is raised with or without preliminary delays, according to its dimensions, and directly sutured to the defect. The raw area left when the flap is raised is closed by direct suture if small, otherwise a split-skin graft is applied. Because of its random vascular pattern its length-breadth ratio is an extremely important limiting factor in design. A 1:1 ratio of length to breadth is the minimum generally tolerable without scrupulous delay and even more favourable ratios like 1:1.5 are preferable.

The direct flap should aim to get as much as possible of the flap in contact with the defect at the initial transfer leaving the minimum to be attached later and a good principle is to make the flap so that any tendency to movement pulls the flap on to the defect rather than away from it. In limb flaps the effect should be to wrap the flap around the limb.

Meticulous planning in reverse is necessary to avoid the tension, kinking and shearing which are so disastrous, and also to ensure that the patient is given as comfortable a position to maintain as possible.

Even in the direct flap there is always a pedicle though it is frequently very short compared with the remainder of the flap. The longer the pedicle the greater the range of permissible mobility of recipient on donor site and the greater the safety factor against tension, etc. On the other hand a long pedicle reduces the length–breadth ratio and in effect narrows the flap from a vascular point of view. Those seeming irreconcilables can both be met on occasion by making the base of the pedicle broader than the segment which is to be inset so that a broad pedicle is combined with a reasonably long one.

Avoidance of raw areas (Fig. 4.13)
The split-skin graft covering the flap donor site is increased in length so that it lines the pedicle segment of the flap where it would otherwise be raw.

Despite the use of these devices greater or smaller raw areas frequently persist and in difficult situations are virtually inevitable.

Division of the flap
An acute angle of fibrous tissue is nearly always built up at the junction of recipient area and flap (Fig. 4.39) so that the flap when divided does not inset naturally into the remaining part of the defect. The flap as a result has to be dissected off the defect and thinned a little, at the same time excising the fibrous tissue of the 'angle' to allow it to sit nicely into the remaining defect. Such dissection, though minimal, does have an adverse effect on the vascular supply and marginal necrosis of the flap is a common result. This can be avoided by detaching the flap completely without attempting an inset. This has the same effect as a delay and while waiting to inset the remainder of the flap in 7 to 10 days, limbs, fingers, etc., can be mobilised as required.

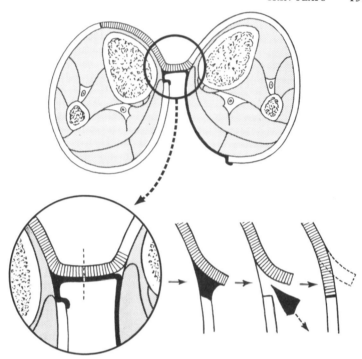

Fig. 4.39 The angle of fibrous tissue usually built up at the junction of the flap and the recipient area which has to be excised to allow the flap to sit into the remainder of the defect. The dissection involved in this has an adverse effect on the blood supply of the flap margin.

PRACTICE OF THE METHOD IN VARIOUS SITES

The upper limb

In major resurfacing of the arm and hand, the usual donor site is the trunk and the flap must be planned so that with the limb in a comfortable position the flap 'wraps round' the limb. In the forearm the limb is most comfortable in the neutral position; extreme pronation or supination is difficult to maintain. Because of this the base of the flap is best made superior where the defect is radial and inferior where the defect is ulnar so that in each case the natural tendency of the limb to move downwards and outwards from the trunk 'wraps' the flap round the recipient site rather than pulling it away from it.

Similar considerations arise in flaps applied to the wrist and dorsum of hand, though on occasion a direct flap from one forearm to the other hand is used and then the broad principles described for cross-leg flaps apply. Cross-arm flaps together with the other types of flap used in Hand Surgery are discussed in detail in chapter 8.

The lower limb
The direct flap used in the leg and foot is the cross-leg flap where the skin of one leg is transferred as a direct flap to cover a defect of the other leg, the appropriate parts of the limbs being approximated by suitable positioning (Fig. 4.40).

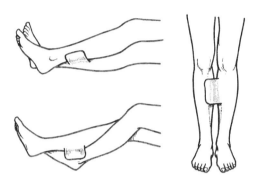

Fig. 4.40 The classical cross-leg flap positions.

The donor sites are limited to:

1. *Middle two-thirds of the length of tibia*. In this segment the site must not include the skin directly over the tibia lest failure of the split-skin graft applied to the secondary defect should leave bare tibia to complicate the transfer. Usually flaps are outlined just behind the subcutaneous surface of tibia based in the direction found to suit best when the procedure is planned.

2. *Lower anterior thigh*. To use this site successfully the defect requiring the flap must be in the vicinity of the heel or ankle (Fig. 4.42c) since in all but the acrobatic these are the only areas capable of ready approximation to the donor site on the thigh. Indeed even with the ankle and heel the position required of the patient takes a degree of agility seldom found in the average adult. The site as a result has very limited usefulness.

In theory a proximally based flap should have a more normally directed vascular flow but in the distally based flap the main direction of the vascular flow remains along the axis of the limb even if reversed in direction and in fact the direction of the base is not of great significance. Disruption of normal flow is likely to be greater in the side-based flap.

Unless the length-breadth ratio is unusually favourable it is advisable to delay cross-leg flaps and the delay can include as a stage elevation of the flap so that perforating veins may be divided. The donor leg of the flap should be avoided as a source of the split-skin graft which covers the secondary defect, for the dressing of the donor site will naturally raise the venous pressure of the leg and such a rise, however small, tends to increase congestion of the flap and helps to set off the cycle of congestion, oedema, kinking, etc., unless extreme care is exercised.

Immobilisation during flap transfer
When a transfer is to the upper limb or head and neck, elastoplast must be relied on in conjunction with sand-bags, pillows, etc., to keep the parts suitably positioned (Fig. 4.41) and the position set up

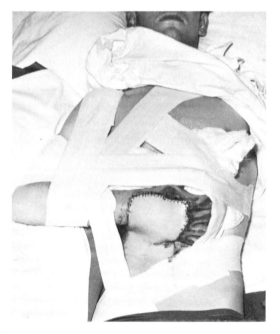

Fig. 4.41 The method of fixing the arm during transfer of a direct flap to the upper limb.

on the operating table has generally to be adjusted when the patient is returned to bed. When the transfer is to the lower limb, whether tube pedicle on the wrist or cross-leg flap, immobilisation by plaster of Paris is much more effective for it takes altogether from the patient the onus of maintaining his position. Plaster does nevertheless impose its own discipline on the surgeon and it must be used with care.

The plaster of Paris can be applied at the time of operation, but prefabrication has undoubted advantages. These procedures, cross-leg flaps especially, are among the more exacting in plastic surgery at all phases—in planning, in execution and in postoperative care. The position of the limbs must be maintained from the moment of inserting the first suture joining flap and recipient site to the final division of the pedicle three to four weeks later. Holding the limbs during suture and subsequent immobilisation is an unrewarding and most fatiguing task. With ample able-bodied assistance, application of the entire plaster cast at the time of operation may be feasible and satisfactory, but when such assistance is minimal all concerned will welcome anything which can speed up the process of postoperative immobilisation. Speeding up is best achieved by prefabricating the plaster cast.

The prefabricated plaster
Prior to the operation, and with the limbs in the position to be maintained postoperatively to permit accurate moulding of the plaster to the muscular contours, lengths of encircling plaster are applied at strategic points so that, strutted together postoperatively (Fig. 4.42), e.g. with lengths of broom-handle, the whole system is held rigidly immobile in its correct position. Added lengths of

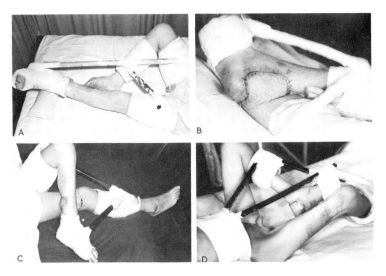

Fig. 4.42 Examples of prefabricated plaster fixation during cross-leg flap transfers.

plaster and struts may be used but seldom are more than three or four needed. The flap is best left exposed while the struts are being applied so that its position can be watched carefully; the slight contamination with plaster has not been significant. In this situation one of the transparent plastic dressings can usefully be employed to protect the suture line.

With a pedicle on the wrist the arm plaster is the really important though most difficult segment of the system and a very carefully applied plaster which includes the hand to the distal transverse crease, well set back from the pedicle inset is used.

The tendency is for the arm to pull from the leg and so slide up the plaster and to prevent this a mean must be sought between the tight plaster which will give rise to swelling and circulatory embarrassment and the slack one which allows movement.

One way of getting round the difficulty is to have the axis of pull of the arm at right angles to the pull of the pedicle. A strong transverse bar incorporated in the plaster across the palm also gives the patient something to grip to prevent sliding.

Joint stiffness

Immobilisation for the three to four weeks which a flap transfer takes is apt to result in joint stiffness. In the young patient this is not of great importance as it clears up very quickly with the removal of the fixation. It is in the older age group that the possibility of permanent limitation of movement has to be taken account of in deciding the pros and cons of using a flap but even there steps can be taken to reduce the possibility very considerably.

The secret of preventing stiffness lies in regular active exercises and the putting of the joints concerned through as full a range of movement as the flap will permit.

When plaster of Paris fixation is used it continues unmodified throughout the three weeks and this is one reason why the method is usually only used in the younger age group where stiffness will only be temporary. In the upper limb and with tube pedicles in general, fixation is progressively relaxed but one does have to accept total immobilisation for the first week or so after transfer of the flap. As soon as the flap is judged to be firmly attached it is extremely important to tell the patient that it is quite safe to pull on the flap in exercising his joints. Patients tend to be very chary of carrying out any movement which creates a feeling of pull on the flap. Active finger exercises are of vital importance in all flaps involving the upper limb and a good physiotherapist is invaluable in making sure that they are carried out.

Just as the patients often complain of discomfort and pain when the joints are fixed they complain of pain when the flap is divided and the full range of joint movements is being restored. These pains tend to persist until a full range is achieved and their presence indicates a need to persist with active exercises rather than discontinue them, a need for reassurance and not rest.

THE TUBE PEDICLE

This is a bipedicled flap which when raised is turned in on itself to form a tube (Fig. 4.43). It is usually raised on the torso for transfer either to the head and neck or one of the limbs.

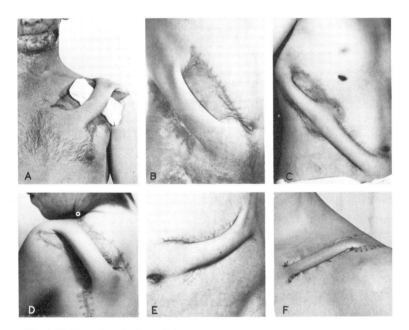

Fig. 4.43 Examples of tube pedicles.
A Acromiopectoral tube.
B Abdominal tube.
C Double abdominal tube with connecting bridge ready for tubing to complete the long tube pedicle.
D Tube pedicle of scapular region. The unusual site was chosen to correct a postburn contracture of neck because the usual sites had sustained full thickness skin loss burning.
E Abdominal tube of unusual direction to be inset into the hand. The direction was chosen to suit positioning of the hand during insetting.
F Clavicular tube pedicle.

Once raised and tubed, the pedicle is left to mature for six weeks during which time the axial vascular re-orientation already described is developed. To give a good start to axial redeployment the tube is placed along a line of venous orientation where possible. The vascular link across the mid-line of the trunk is poor and it is seldom wise to construct a flap which crosses this line. The **abdominal tube pedicle** usually uses the thoraco-epigastric venous axis and the limiting length-breadth ratio is generally assessed at $2\frac{1}{2}$:1. If more length is required two tubes of standard length with a connecting bridge may be constructed. In due course the bridge is delayed along its margins, raised and finally tubed to complete the 'double' tube. On the chest the **acromiopectoral tube pedicle** is used particularly in the male and lying as it does on a most efficient venous pathway a 3:1 ratio of length to breadth is quite safe.

In most instances the tube pedicle is a random vascular pattern flap. Although it is probable that an axial pattern is sometimes inadvertently incorporated this is purely fortuitous and management of tube pedicles in general is based on the assumption that the pattern is initially random. The only approximation to a concession in conscious planning to providing an axial pattern is the designing of the tube along a line of venous orientation where possible.

Vascular pressure measurements in tube pedicles have shown that although the pressure at both ends is usually equal there is sometimes a striking vascular pressure gradient along the tube with the pressure at one end much higher. Such dominance of one end is the result of accidentally incorporating an artery at one end and creating in effect an axial pattern flap. Detachment of the arterial end produces a sudden and profound change in vascular dynamics which can be disastrous and result in local necrosis when detachment is coupled with movement of the tube. This explains the unexpected necrosis when the sternal end of an acromiopectoral tube is divided and the flap transferred, for elevation of the sternal attachment has cut off one or more of the perforating arteries of the internal mammary system. Similar problems can affect the abdominal tube which has incorporated the superficial epigastric arteriovenous system by accident.

The abdominal tube pedicle is most often carried on the wrist; the acromiopectoral tube pedicle, with the surge of popularity of the deltopectoral flap, is rarely used. It is waltzed on its shoulder attachment.

A tube pedicle may also be used as a carrier for a 'pancake' flap or 'spade' (Fig. 4.8) delayed on to one end; such a flap must be most carefully delayed in stages.

The alternative sites for tubes (e.g. Fig. 4.43) are used much less commonly, mainly when the usual sites are not available because of scarring, etc.

Six weeks must be allowed to elapse between the raising of a tube pedicle and the next stage of the transfer, and if there is a suspicion that the pedicle to be divided is a dominant one, a delay is advisable. It is certainly wise with the medial end of an acromiopectoral tube pedicle so frequently is an artery present.

The technique of transfer to a carrier has been described (p. 124). The remaining stages are of transfer on the carrier and completing the transfer.

Transfer on the carrier (Fig. 4.44)
This is essentially similar to the wrist inset. After severing the remaining abdominal attachment the flap is moved on its carrier to

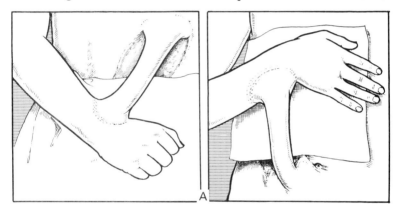

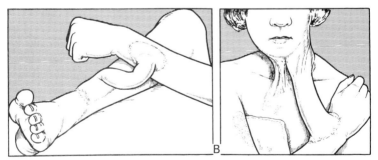

Fig. 4.44 Steps in the transfer of abdominal tube pedicles.
A   Attachment to wrist carriers showing radial and ulnar attachments.
B   Transfer on wrist carriers.
Note in each case the large segment inset to provide a vascular attachment adequate for the next transfer.

be inset into part or all of its destination. It is not usual to aim at final disposition of the flap on the recipient area at this stage. What is aimed at rather is attachment of the free end of the tube to a suitable segment of the recipient area having regard to the need to establish a vascular link-up adequate to nourish the flap when it is later detached from the wrist to be completely untubed and inset. It is therefore advisable to give the flap as big an attachment as is expedient with positioning of the wrist, etc. To increase the raw area of the flap the tube is undone as far as required excising the scar of the tubing and thinning appropriately. The raw area is measured against the selected segment of the recipient site and an appropriate area of skin is excised. Where possible a small trapdoor flap can be raised from the recipient site to close off the raw area where tubing of the flap begins again.

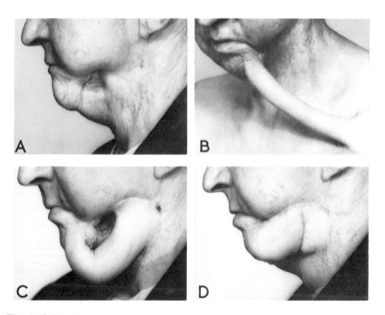

Fig. 4.45 Double attachment of a tube pedicle prior to final insetting. Closure of fistula (A) by acromiopectoral tube inset into a reception area (B) immediately anterior to the fistula. The double attachment is made by insetting the other end (C) immediately posterior to the fistula prior to untubing and closure of the defect (D).

Completing the transfer

After a further period of three weeks the pedicle is removed from the wrist, the scar of the tubing is excised, and the flap is opened. It is found on opening the tube that an axial line of scarring has developed along its centre which prevents it from untubing readily. With the tube partially opened, it gives the appearance of a well-defined layer like deep fascia and only excision, or at very least, deep multiple longitudinal scoring of this layer will permit the flap to untube completely and spread to its original dimensions. When the flap is spread out and thinned if necessary, the amount of skin to be excised is defined and removed so that the flap can be sutured in position. It is not always safe to complete the transfer and spread the whole pedicle in a single procedure. The detached wrist inset may then be set into its final destination leaving the still tubed central segment of the pedicle (Fig. 4.45) to be untubed and inset three weeks or so later once both ends have an efficient vascular attachment.

The wrist trapdoor is sutured back in its original position. It is less easy to return to its original situation that one might expect, for the trapdoor will be found to have 'shrunk' somewhat and the several wound edges have to be mobilised to achieve closure. A good suture line is often difficult to get, but in this time fortunately works wonders in most cases.

5

Muscle and myocutaneous flaps

MUSCLE FLAPS

The principle of moving a muscle to cover a surface which is unsuitable for skin grafting in order to convert it into one which will accept a skin graft is now well established. The technique is most often and most effectively used in covering bare cortical bone and open joint and the tissue transfer is referred to as a **muscle flap**. The surface is covered by the highly vascular muscle belly and on top of this the skin graft is applied. The value of the method lies in the fact that it allows such defects to be resurfaced with skin without recourse to skin flaps.

Muscle flaps are rarely needed in the upper limb because convenient and effective alternative reconstructive techniques already exist. In the lower limb the situation is quite different. The alternatives available such as cross-leg flaps or other distant flaps have been sufficiently unsatisfactory to encourage the development of alternatives such as muscle flaps. The need also arises more often in the lower limb. The tibia with its extensive subcutaneous surface is the bone most often requiring cover; the joint most often exposed, open and in urgent need of skin cover, is the knee.

The muscles which have been used with greatest effect are **gastrocnemius** and **soleus**. Each head of gastrocnemius has its own neurovascular hilum close to its origin and the muscle bellies remain separate until they insert into an aponeurosis, common to both, on their deep surface (Fig. 5.1). Soleus has an origin which spans the upper tibia and fibula but its neurovascular hilum is also close to its origin (Fig. 5.1). Its superficial surface is covered by an aponeurosis in its lower part. The aponeuroses covering the opposed surfaces of gastrocnemius and soleus, though in contact with one another, are quite separate until they fuse below to form the tendo Achillis.

These anatomical features make it possible to dissect any one of the three muscle bellies free of the others, divide its distal attachment, mobilise it towards its origin and swing it medially or laterally, using its neurovascular pedicle as a pivot point. The medial

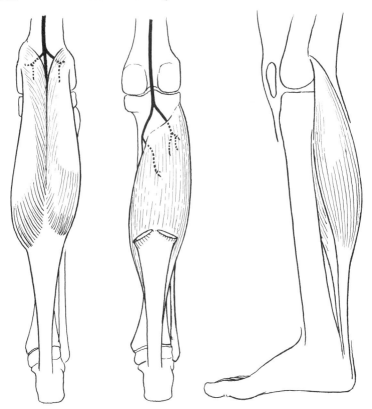

Fig. 5.1 Anatomical features of gastrocnemius and soleus and their dominant vascular hila.

head of gastrocnemius is capable of reaching the upper third of the medial aspect of the tibia and the corresponding portion of the knee joint. The lateral head, less often required, can cover the upper fibula and lateral aspect of the knee joint. Soleus, moved medially, can cover the central half of the tibial shaft.

Certain points of technique are common to all muscle flaps and they are also peculiar to muscle flaps. They require to be observed scrupulously if satisfactory results are to be achieved consistently.

Any transfer of muscle must be without tension if the blood supply of the muscle is not to be compromised. Embarrassment of circulation shows in the appearance of the muscle fibres, with slight darkening in colour where the blood supply is inadequate. Allowance needs to be made in planning for a degree of swelling of the muscle belly in the early phase following transfer. The need to avoid tension means that tunnelling of the muscle through deep fascia or under skin to reach its destination is unwise as a rule. In the lower limb the deep fascia is strong and unyielding and in practice tension is likely to arise more often from it than from skin. There should be no hesitation in dividing the fascia widely, and even excising areas if necessary, to eliminate tension. Skin bridges over the flap should also be divided.

Muscle does not tolerate sutures which exert significant tension. Any sutures through muscle fibre should be only of a tacking nature, used to hold the muscle over the defect without exerting traction. Associated aponeurosis or tendon should be used wherever possible for holding sutures. It is for this purpose that a fringe of tendon is taken with the muscle belly when the muscle is detached distally.

The flap of muscle covering the bony or joint surface is covered in turn by a split-skin graft. Immediate grafting can be used; alternatively a delayed graft can be applied. In either event exposed grafting is preferable because no pressure is then applied to the muscle bed.

In the case of an acute injury the skin incisions required for exposure, mobilisation and transfer of the muscle are usually dictated by the site and size of the exposed bone and/or open joint and any associated skin loss. In the absence of clear-cut indications, gastrocnemius can be exposed by an incision in the lower popliteal fossa curving downwards and medially or laterally according to the muscle belly to be used. Soleus can be exposed along its medial border using a vertical incision parallel to and approximately 2 cm behind the posterior border of the subcutaneous tibial surface.

Gastrocnemius is easily separated from soleus using finger dissection and the line between its two muscle bellies is readily felt through the aponeurosis which covers its deep surface and holds the bellies together. Mobilised deeply as far as the tendo Achillis the insertion of the particular muscle belly can be divided leaving a fringe of tendon on the muscle. Splitting of the aponeurosis on the deep surface in a proximal direction allows the muscle belly to be mobilised towards the popliteal fossa as far as required (Fig. 5.2).

Soleus in addition to being readily separated from gastrocnemius has a good cleavage plane deeply, between the muscle and the posterior tibial vessels and nerves though several veins entering its deep surface may require ligation and division before the muscle can be mobilised. Division distally with a fringe of tendo Achillis allows the muscle to be mobilised along each border, dividing deep fascia as required, until it can be swung medially to cover the tibia (Fig. 5.3).

A little extra cover of the tibia below the reach of soleus can be obtained if the tendon of flexor digitorum longus is divided and the muscle is brought round alongside soleus. Mobilisation of this

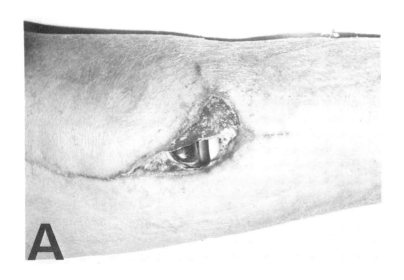

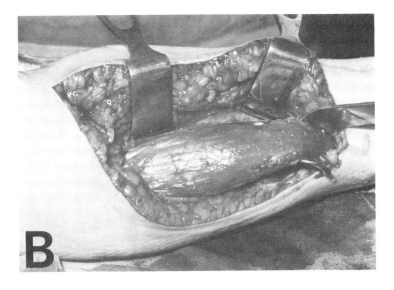

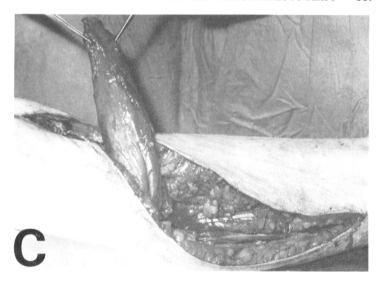

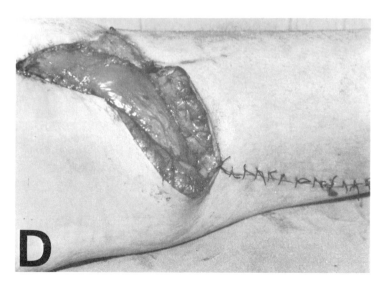

Fig. 5.2 Use of gastrocnemius muscle flap to close open knee joint in a patient with severe rheumatoid arthritis, following postoperative wound breakdown and exposure of a joint replacement prosthesis.

A   Open knee joint with prosthesis visible.
B   Medial belly of gastrocnemius exposed.
C   Muscle belly divided at insertion into tendo Achillis and swung upwards to cover knee defect.
D   Muscle sutured into knee defect with direct closure of secondary defect.

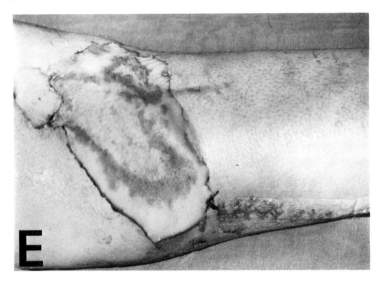

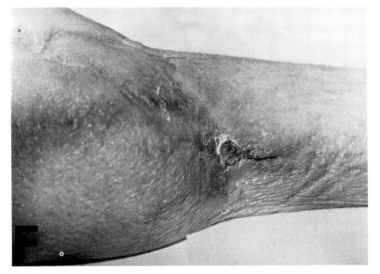

Fig. 5.2 (*cont.*)
E   Delayed exposed graft covering the muscle flap, showing take over of the muscle.
F   End result, showing knee defect closed.

muscle must be carried out with great care to avoid injuring its neurovascular bundle which enters the middle third of the muscle.

The functional deficit which results from use of these muscle flaps is made up quite quickly by the other muscles of the flexor compartment.

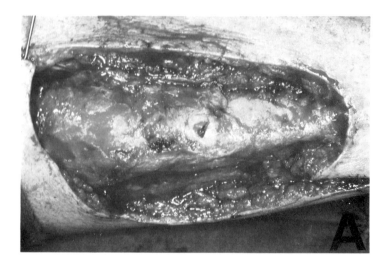

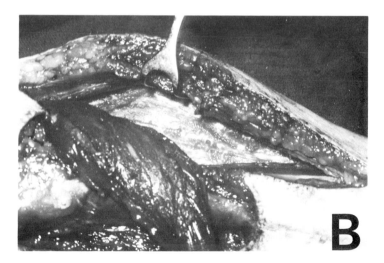

Fig. 5.3 Use of soleus muscle flap to cover bare tibia.
A   Defect, showing mixture of soft tissue, tibia covered with periosteum and area of bare tibia with central sinus.
B   Gastrocnemius retracted, soleus muscle divided at insertion into tendo Achillis and swung medially to cover the area of bare bone.

Other muscles which have been used as flaps are flexor hallucis longus for small defects of the medial aspect of the ankle and extensores digitorum longus and hallucis longus for defects of the anterior tibia. None of these sources compare even remotely for worth with gastrocnemius and soleus.

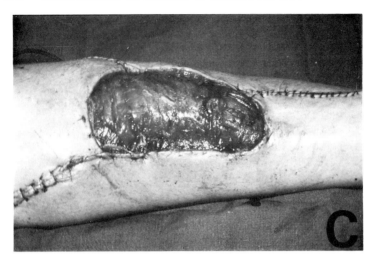

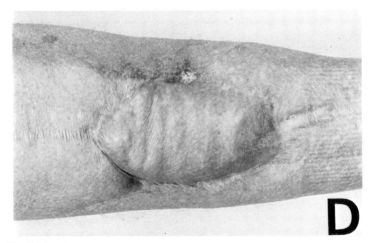

Fig. 5.3 (*cont.*)
C Defect left after suture of skin incisions showing base of muscle and other surfaces suitable for grafting.
D The end result.

MYOCUTANEOUS FLAPS

An extension of muscle flaps which has considerably increased their therapeutic potential has been the idea of transferring a muscle together with the skin overlying it in the form of a composite **myocutaneous flap**. In such a transfer the skin element is perfused through its vascular connections with the underlying muscle.

When our knowledge of the vascular behaviour of skin flaps is considered together with recently acquired knowledge of how myocutaneous flaps behave it is apparent that skin derives its blood supply from more than one source. The branches given off by the major vessels at the root of the limbs, the anastomoses around the joints, and vessels derived from the segmental perforating systems are the vessels which sustain skin flaps as discussed in chapter 4. The successful use of myocutaneous flaps has demonstrated that these vessels are reinforced by vascular connections between the skin and the underlying muscles. The contribution which each makes to the circulation through intact skin is not known but the important practical point has been established empirically that certain areas of skin are capable of surviving on the blood supply which they derive from the muscle immediately deep, even if other sources are markedly reduced and even on occasion cut off completely.

Certain muscles, as the use of muscle flaps has demonstrated, receive their blood supply via a localised neurovascular hilum and can be moved using this hilum as a pivot point. These muscles are the potential sources of myocutaneous flaps. Of the many possible myocutaneous flaps the ones used in practice are those which fill a therapeutic need and are simple to use, which are found most reliable and safe, and which leave the minimum of disability from loss of function of the muscle component. The flaps which most strikingly fulfil these criteria are the **latissimus dorsi flap**, the **tensor fasciae latae flap**, the **pectoralis major flap**, the **gastrocnemius flap** and the **gracilis flap**.

Confidence in the ability of the skin element of the myocutaneous flap to rely absolutely on the underlying muscle for its blood supply has been carried in certain of the flaps to the extent of making its dependence total by converting the skin component into an island. The geometry of the transfer may make this essential but it should not be made a routine. These flaps, like all flaps, have a failure rate though they have not as yet been used sufficiently widely for this to be documented in a definitive manner. To wantonly cut off any additional blood supply reaching the skin by other routes is foolish.

The attachment between the skin and the muscle is not always a strong one and it is a safeguard when the composite flap is being raised to tack the muscle to the skin with sutures to prevent the possible adverse effect of shearing strain on the blood vessels passing between the two.

Latissimus dorsi flap

Latissimus dorsi is a large, flat muscle whose blood supply, from the subscapular vessels, arises in the axilla close to its tendon of insertion, arborising on the deep surface of the muscle (Fig. 5.4). The skin component of the flap overlies the muscle. The composite transfer was originally used to resurface the anterolateral chest wall and has clearly a useful role in the wake of post-mastectomy, post-radiational problems. It is also available for cover of the axilla (Fig. 5.5) and upper arm.

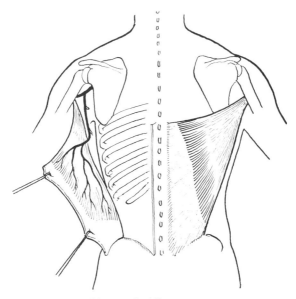

Fig. 5.4 Latissimus dorsi and its vascular hilum.

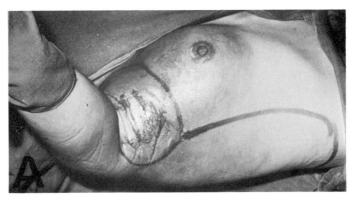

Fig. 5.5 Use of latissimus dorsi myocutaneous flap to cover axillary defect.
A   Initial condition, mixed radiation damage and residual tumour of axilla, showing area to be excised and skin element of latissimus dorsi flap outlined.

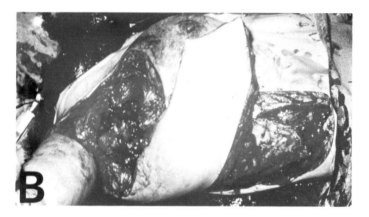

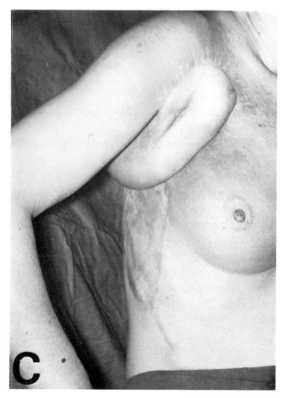

B   Excision completed, flap raised and in process of being transposed into the defect.
C   Transfer completed with split-skin grafting of secondary defect.

The anterior border of the muscle belly runs approximately vertically down over the lateral chest wall towards the iliac crest from the pivot point of the flap near the tendon of insertion. Measurements are made from this area in designing the flap and in view of the lack of precision in siting the point on the surface and the fact that the flap is frequently passing round the convexity, generosity in estimating its desirable length is a wise precaution. The anterior border of the skin element of the flap can extend up to 5 cm in front of the muscle border, the overlap being in the nature of a 'random' addition. The length and breadth of the flap are determined by the geometry of the transfer. Transfer with the flap extended as far as the iliac crest without necrosis has been described.

In raising the flap the anterior border of the muscle is defined and the plane deep to it is established over much of the extent of the tissue to be transferred, visualising the vessels and being careful not to damage them. The entire composite flap is then raised and, mobilised proximally as far as necessary, is transferred into the defect. It is stated that the defect can usually be closed by direct suture but this will clearly depend on the breadth of the flap. There need be no hesitation in grafting the secondary defect instead, by delayed grafting if need be.

Tensor fasciae latae flap

In the lateral aspect of the thigh the fascia lata is markedly thickened to form the iliotibial tract, receiving into its upper part the insertions of gluteus maximus behind and tensor fasciae latae further forward (Fig. 5.6). As the tract passes distally it overlies vastus lateralis but there is no attachment between the two structures. Although the fascia lata encircles the thigh the thickening which constitutes the iliotibial tract virtually ceases along a line dropped vertically from the anterior superior iliac spine.

The tensor fasciae latae receives a blood supply in its lower part from the lateral femoral circumflex vessels which reaches it about the level of the pubic tubercle. This supply appears to extend into the upper two-thirds of the tract.

The tensor fasciae latae myocutaneous flap is superiorly based on the lateral aspect of the thigh and makes use of the iliotibial tract as its 'muscle' element. Its anterior border runs vertically along a line brought just lateral to the anterior superior iliac spine in order to avoid the lateral cutaneous nerve of thigh. Its posterior border approximates to the line running down from the greater trochanter. The length of the flap is determined by the geometry of the transfer but it can safely extend to the junction between the upper two-thirds

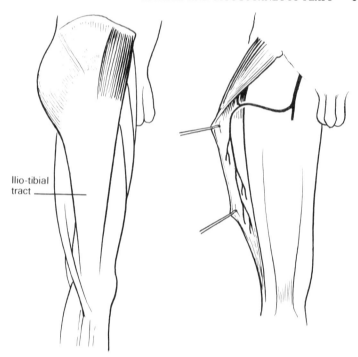

Fig. 5.6 Anatomical features and vascular hilum of tensor fasciae latae.

and the lower third of the thigh. The flap is technically extremely easy to raise because the plane between the tract and vastus lateralis is so well defined and avascular. It can be raised proximally to the level of the pubic tubercle. Transposition thereafter can be anterior or posterior depending on the site of the defect, e.g. groin, trochanter, ischium. The secondary defect is split-skin grafted (Fig. 5.7).

Pectoralis major flap
The fibres of pectoralis major converge like a fan from its extensive origin along the margins of the anterior chest wall towards the anterior axillary fold. Its main artery of supply is the pectoral branch of the acromiothoracic axis. This vessel reaches the deep surface of the muscle just medial to the tendon of pectoralis minor near its origin from the coracoid process. Together with its accompanying veins the artery then arborises over the deep surface of the muscle in a generally downward and medial direction, cutting across the line of many of the fibres of the muscle in the process. It is this arteriovenous system which provides the vascular basis of the pectoralis major myocutaneous flap (Fig. 5.8).

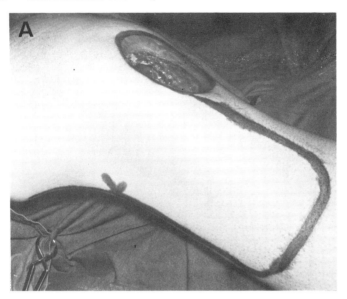

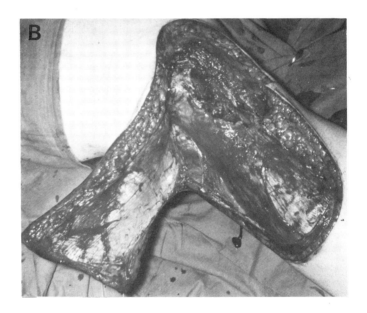

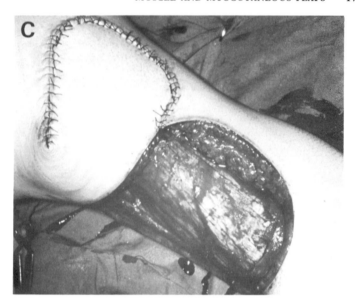

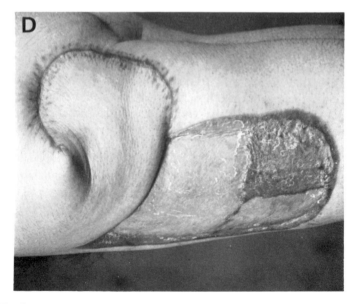

Fig. 5.7 Use of tensor fasciae latae myocutaneous flap to cover defect overlying the greater trochanter in a non-paraplegic.

A   The defect and the tensor fasciae latae flap outlined.

B   The flap raised, showing incorporation of iliotibial tract in the flap substance.

C   The flap transposed and sutured to the defect.

D   The flap healed in position and the secondary defect split-skin grafted.

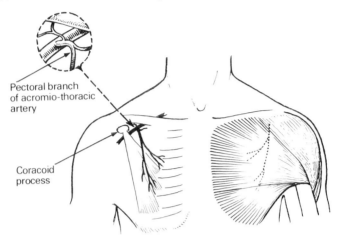

Pectoral branch
of acromio-thoracic
artery

Coracoid
process

Fig. 5.8 The vascular basis of the pectoralis major myocutaneous flap, showing the pectoral branch of the acromiothoracic artery arising immediately medial to the coracoid process and running downwards and medially between pectoralis major and pectoralis minor.

The flap has been used both with a composite pedicle of skin and underlying muscle and as an island of skin with a pedicle of muscle alone. The skin which is transferred when the flap is used as an island lies below and medial to the nipple about the level of the 6th rib. The available skin in this site which directly overlies pectoralis major is quite small in area but it can safely be extended beyond the actual muscle on to the aponeurosis covering the anterior abdomen for at least 4 cm. When the flap is used as a composite skin-muscle transfer it can be similarly extended.

If a composite skin-muscle pedicle is used the parallel lines of the skin flap are centred on the coracoid process which can be felt just below the clavicle. Commencing at the level of the clavicle the lines pass downwards and medially to the skin site described above. In raising the flap the skin incisions are deepened to section the muscle fibres in the same lines as the skin.

If an island myocutaneous flap is used (Fig. 5.9) the area of skin to be transferred is outlined and incised around its margin deeply to muscle or aponeurosis. The muscle which is to provide its pedicle is then exposed. The incision used to expose the muscle must obviously begin above just medial to the coronoid process. It must also end below on the incision encircling the skin island, preferably near its most proximal point. Between these points its course may vary, depending on such matters as coincident or previous use of a

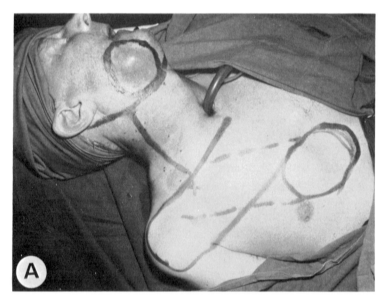

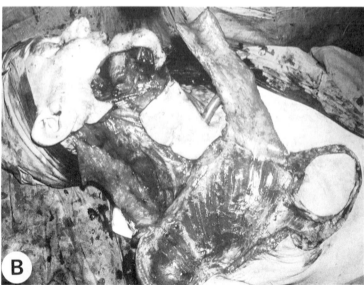

Fig. 5.9 Use of pectoralis major myocutaneous flap to reconstruct the intra-oral component of the full-thickness defect created by resection of cheek and mandible in continuity with a radical neck dissection for squamous carcinoma of lower alveolus. A simultaneous deltopectoral flap was used to provide skin cover. *The simultaneous use of the two flaps demonstrates the independence of their vascular basis.*
A The defect outlined and the two flaps, pectoralis major island myocutaneous and deltopectoral, marked out on the skin.
B Resection and radical neck dissection completed and deltopectoral flap raised exposing pectoralis major. Skin island of pectoralis major flap outlined by skin incision.

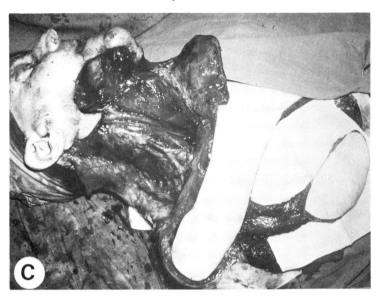

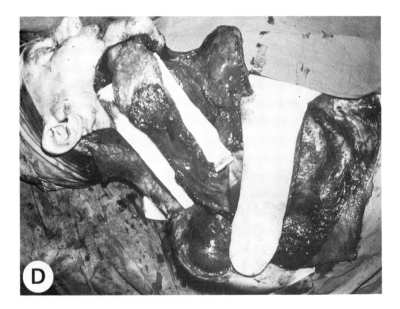

Fig. 5.9 (*cont.*)

C   Pedicles of both flaps demonstrated after elevation.

D   Pectoralis major flap transposed into intra-oral defect. The pectoral branch of the acromiothoracic axis can be seen running over the muscle pedicle along its axial line. The area of flap beyond the muscle can be seen.

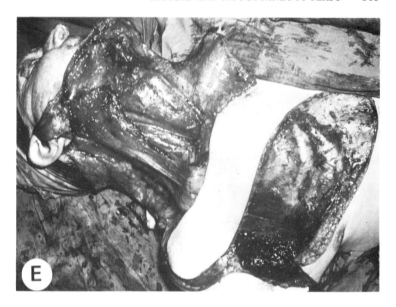

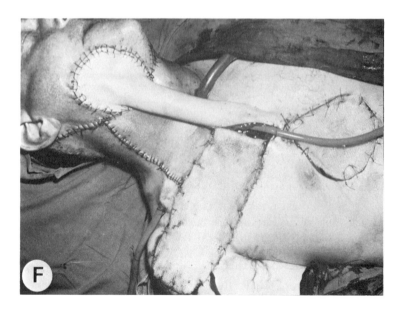

E   Pectoralis major flap sutured in position showing how the muscle pedicle covers
    the carotid arteries around and above the bifurcation.
F   Transfer of deltopectoral flap to complete reconstruction by providing skin cover.

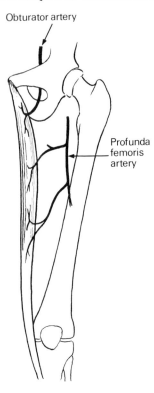

Fig. 5.10 The vascular hila of gracilis showing its segmental character. The hilum derived from the obturator artery is one used when a gracilis myocutaneous flap is raised.

deltopectoral flap or the presence of the breast. The pedicle of muscle is similar to that used when the muscle is combined with skin, as broad as the skin island and extended upwards to the clavicle.

When raised as an island or as a combined skin-muscle flap, the muscle pedicle is carefully elevated off the ribs and intercostal muscles, leaving pectoralis minor behind, upwards almost to the coracoid process, disturbing the hilar vessels as little as possible in the process. It becomes apparent in raising the muscle off the deeper structures that vessels enter from other sources but the arteriovenous system on which the flap is relying appears to be capable of perfusing it adequately. The fact that the incisions into the muscle cut across its fibres inevitably makes construction of the muscle pedicle somewhat lacking in elegance.

If possible the secondary defect is closed by direct suture but split-skin grafting should be used if it is needed.

How far the flap will reach and other aspects of its geometry are established by measurement from the vascular hilum which is its pivot point. Its main uses are in resurfacing defects of the lower face and neck, and in intra-oral reconstruction. In this latter role, when a radical neck dissection in continuity has been carried out an incidental bonus provided by the flap is its ability to cover and protect the major vessels, a considerable virtue particularly when the neck has been previously irradiated. An obviously limiting factor in its usage may be the hairy male chest and the presence of the breast in the female may also call for modifications of design.

Gastrocnemius flap

The virtues of the muscle element of this flap used by itself have already been stressed but its therapeutic possibilities have been extended a little by incorporating the overlying skin. Like the muscle flap from which it is derived the myocutaneous flap may be medial or lateral. The skin element can be extended beyond the muscle, a little on each side and distally as far as half-way between the distal insertion of the muscle belly and the corresponding

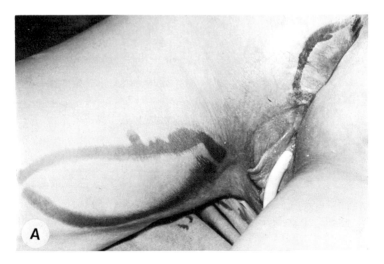

Fig. 5.11 Use of gracilis myocutaneous flap to close a urinary fistula just below the coccyx which has followed an excision of rectum.
A The defect which will be prepared to receive the gracilis flap and the gracilis myocutaneous flap have been outlined. The line drawn between the pubic tubercle to the hamstring insertion on the tibia, used to locate the position of gracilis is visible.

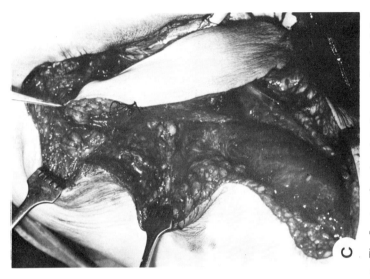

C   The flap transferred ready to be sutured to the defect.

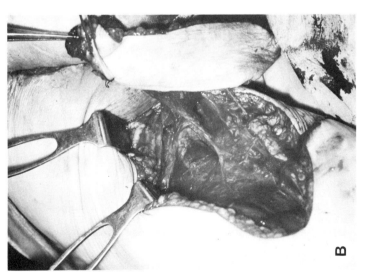

B   The flap raised with the vascular pedicle defined.

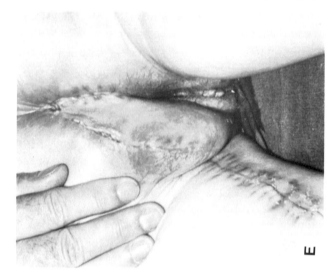

E   The final result.

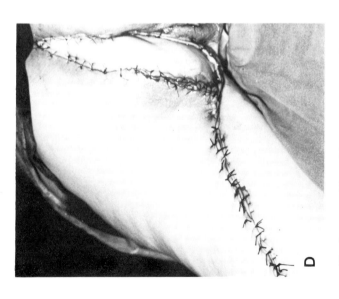

D   The flap sutured in position and secondary defect closed by direct suture.

malleolus. It is this distal extension which may make the flap preferable to the muscle flap alone, increasing its reach and making it possible to extend its role even into that of a cross-leg myocutaneous flap and resurface the opposite leg.

Gracilis flap

As a muscle source gracilis has the virtue that its loss creates no disability. It has several segmental vascular sources but the one used as the hilum on which the flap will pivot is approximately 7 cm below the pubic tubercle, somewhat less than one third of the way down the muscle (Fig. 5.10)

The anterior extent of the skin element of the flap lies behind the line from the pubic tubercle to the ham-string insertion on the tibia and the muscle itself lies behind adductor longus, this muscle being used in identifying both gracilis and the anterior dissection plane between it and the adductor muscles, longus and brevis. It is from between these two muscles that the vascular pedicle emerges.

Once gracilis has been identified the skin flap can be centred on it usually in the form of an elliptical island (Fig. 5.11). The use of an island in this way adds considerably to the reach of the flap and indeed is largely unavoidable if it is to have any worthwhile versatility. The proximal tip of the island extends almost to the origin of the muscle from the ischiopubic ramus; distally it can extend to mid-thigh. The distal part of the flap is its most vulnerable part because the underlying muscle at this point is receiving blood from a more distal segmental source.

The flap can be used to cover defects of the perineum, pubis, ischial fossa and groin area.

PART TWO

Surgical applications

6

General surgery

The need for plastic surgical methods in general surgery arises in many different ways and the only factor common to all is that skin requires to be replaced. Skin loss may have resulted from the pathological process itself, from the surgical attack on it, or from a combination of both. Consideration of the various ways in which the need for repair arises will be concerned particularly with the influence of the pathological condition on the surgeon's approach and how it dictates the type of repair necessary.

A few miscellaneous conditions defy classification but most examples of skin injury or loss requiring replacement fall into the broad categories of **traumatic, infective** and **postsurgical.**

TRAUMATIC SKIN LOSS

Trauma can be **thermal, mechanical** and **radiational.** It is not proposed to discuss thermal trauma as a separate entity for an adequate discussion would entail consideration of aspects outwith the scope of this book but much of the discussion on the granulating area and its skin cover is directly applicable to the care of a full-thickness skin loss burn.

MECHANICAL TRAUMA

Mechanical injury may denude any skin area but the parts particularly prone to injury of this type are the *scalp*, the *limbs* and the *scrotum*.

The scalp
The usual mechanism, less common with a more widespread use of suitable hair-enclosing caps in industry, is for the hair to be caught in machinery avulsing part or all of the scalp. The avulsed segment may be partially or completely avulsed.

If only **partly avulsed** the flap should be preserved and sutured back in position after suitable toilet, shaving, etc., no matter how small its pedicle. Retained in this way it can be watched until a line demarcating viable flap from slough is established. Much more of the flap may survive than the size of its pedicle might have suggested. Once demarcated the slough can be excised while it is dry and relatively sterile. Excision can be followed by the application of an immediate split-skin graft, failing which closely set sheets of skin can be applied 4 or 5 days later. The main contra-indication to the immediate graft is the inclusion of the pericranium in the avulsed flap; the treatment of this complication is described below.

When the segment has been **completely avulsed** it should under no circumstances be sutured back in position. There is no prospect of such a free graft taking and the optimism of the surgeon watching and hoping will only delay the removal of the inevitable slough.

Treatment depends on the plane of avulsion. The usual plane of cleavage is through the loose areolar tissue deep to the galaea aponeurotica and the pericranium which this leaves intact makes an excellent bed for graft. It should be completely covered with split-skin sheet grafts as a primary measure (Fig. 6.1). The scalp is an ideal site for the use of exposed grafting. If for any reason the graft cannot be applied straightaway it is advisable to dress the pericranium with care so that it does not get the chance to become

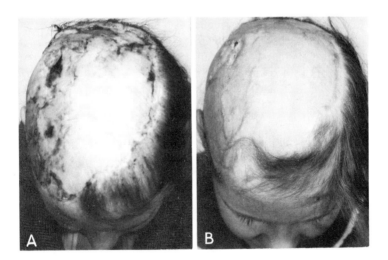

Fig. 6.1 Immediate cover with split-skin grafts following scalp avulsion when the pericranium is intact, showing the rapidity of healing.
A Appearance two weeks after injury.
B Seven weeks after injury showing complete healing.

dry and necrotic. It is at this early stage, before it has granulated, that the pericranium, left exposed, can so easily become mummified. When the forehead is involved, the smooth, uniformly thick graft of the dermatome gives the best cosmetic result. It can be applied either as a primary procedure or secondarily after excising the primary graft (Fig. 6.2).

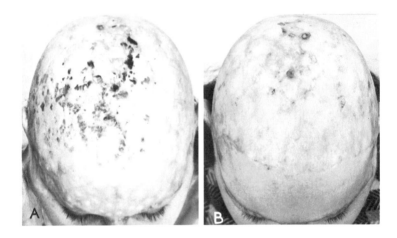

Fig. 6.2 Use of a dermatome split-skin graft in secondary replacement of forehead skin when the cosmetic result of the primary graft is unsatisfactory.

A   The poor cosmetic result of pinch grafts applied primarily.
B   Replacement with the dermatome graft.

More rarely the skull is either partly or completely denuded of pericranium over the area of avulsion and treatment of the bare area of skull becomes quite different, more tedious and difficult. Bare outer table of skull will not take a graft and methods have to be adopted to produce 'bleeding bone' which will granulate (Fig. 6.3). The fastest and surest way of getting the bone to granulate is to chisel away the outer table of skull. With experience an immediate split-skin graft can be got to take on such a surface but little is lost by waiting until reasonable granulations have developed. Chiselling has frequently to be repeated as small areas fail to granulate. The whole procedure is extremely tedious for both patient and surgeon. The end result, too, is much less satisfactory as the lack of mobility and cushioning under the graft make it susceptible to minor trauma.

No hair grows from the avulsed area and this may call for subsequent surgery. The position can sometimes be improved by moving a flap of any remaining normal scalp to the front of the scalp

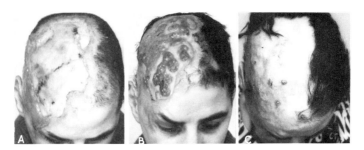

Fig. 6.3 Healing following destruction of the pericranium. In this example destruction was by burning but the sequence of events is similar whe the skull is exposed by avulsion of the scalp.

A Bare outer table of skull.
B Patchy granulations 4 months later.
C State of healing 13 months after A showing areas of instability.

to provide an anterior hair-line. The hair growing back from such a flap brushed appropriately can cover the bald area and though never quite natural gives a better result than many wigs.

The limbs

Extensive loss of skin from a limb is most often the result of a wringer or roller injury which causes degloving.

The usual cause is either the catching of a limb in power driven rollers, e.g. the wringer of a washing machine, or the running over of a limb by a pneumatic tyre, both of which produce a sudden severe shearing strain (Fig. 6.4). The results differ only in severity. Bony or joint injury may be associated, and the management of such a mixed injury is discussed on page 220, but the characteristic feature is the flaying of the skin. The word 'flaying' must be qualified for it may be **anatomical** or **physiological**. If anatomically flayed, the skin is actually torn off; if physiologically, the skin surface is intact but there is complete disruption at the level of the deep fascia with undermining. At the same time the vascular network of the skin is damaged more or less severely by the sudden extreme tension set up by the shearing strain, usually severely enough to cause ischaemic necrosis of skin and superficial fascia.

It must be realised that initially there may be little evidence clinically of the severity or extent of the vascular and skin damage—unless it is tested for. The clinical sign to be looked for in such an injury is failure of the skin to blanch when pressed with return of colour when the pressure is released or, when a skin edge is present, absence of dermal bleeding. Both signs indicate absence of

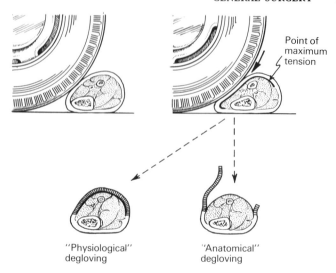

"Physiological"
degloving

"Anatomical"
degloving

Fig. 6.4 The mechanism of degloving.

active skin circulation. Over the whole undermined area the skin must be regarded as suspect and the surgeon must decide what is viable and can be saved, or dead and to be excised. It is positive evidence of circulation which decides viability and if there is not positive evidence of viability the skin should be excised. A clearer picture of the skin area which retains an active circulation can sometimes be obtained by observing the distribution of the reactive hyperaemia which develops when a sphygmomanometer placed proximal to the injured segment is released after being left inflated for five minutes—the **tourniquet test**.

Here as in the scalp early grafting should be carried out (Fig. 6.5). Although the general condition may overshadow the local and dictate at least temporary delay a local assessment should be made as soon as possible, the non-viable skin being excised and the resulting defect split-skin grafted after suitable debridement if necessary. As much skin as possible should be applied with priority to the flexures and areas with underlying tendons.

Damage to muscle is often present and excision of necrotic tissue must be as radical as is consistent with the preservation of such vital structures as arteries and nerves. Only on a healthy base will a graft take and residual necrotic tissue will mean graft failure.

It is not unusual for at least part of the avulsed skin to be relatively undamaged and such skin can be re-applied as a whole skin graft to the debrided surface after all its subcutaneous fat has been carefully

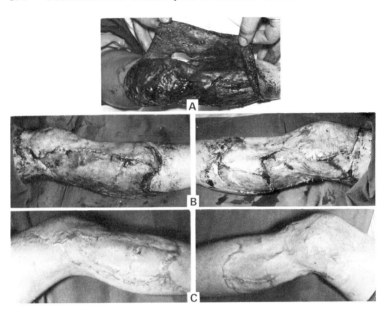

Fig. 6.5 Degloving of leg primarily resurfaced with sheet split-skin grafts.

A Extent of injury.
B First dressing seven days later.
C Healing with full function.

excised. The Gibson Ross dermatome* has been used to cut a very thick split-skin graft from the degloved tissue and is extremely effective in this role. The ultimate result when such a graft is successfully used is significantly better than that of a split-skin graft cut from elsewhere.

Above, all things should not be allowed to drift until the slough separates slowly and spontaneously. If the injury has not been recognised primarily and only becomes obvious when a slough forms, the slough should be excised as soon as demarcated and the area grafted. To wait beyond this is to wait for the infection, mess and delay of slough separation with consequent grafting difficulties.

The scrotum

The catching up of the scrotal skin with the trousers on a horizontally rotating shaft is the usual cause of avulsion of the scrotum. In the past the denuded testicles were implanted in the thighs or

---

* Gibson, T. and Ross, D. S. Dermatome for preparing large skin grafts from detached skin and fat. *Lancet* 1965; i: 252–3. Available from Chas. F. Thackray & Sons, Leeds.

covered by a flap but it has been shown that they can be covered with a free skin graft. Often the avulsed skin is available and relatively undamaged and it has been successfully used as a whole skin graft after careful excision of the dartos muscle layer. As an alternative the use of split-skin graft has been described.

These techniques should only be used by an expert; success calls for experience and skill. Such cases should be referred to a plastic surgery unit in the first instance.

RADIATIONAL TRAUMA

The forms of radiational trauma which may call for plastic surgical methods are **radionecrosis** and **radiodermatitis**. These conditions are late results of irradiation (Fig. 6.6) and many of the worst examples are seen in patients treated inexpertly for conditions in which radiotherapy has either long since been abandoned as a therapeutic measure or in which the actual method of treatment has been radically modified, as for example in thyrotoxicosis, tuberculous cervical adenitis, sycosis barbae, acne vulgaris, lupus vulgaris, haemangioma and many others.

With a greater awareness of the dangers of radiation and more expert use of the various techniques these late complications are less common but they still do occur even in the most careful hands. The area particularly prone to develop radionecrosis or radiodermatitis sufficiently severely to merit treatment is the oral cavity and its environs when a carcinoma has been treated by radiotherapy. The ear and the postmastectomy scar are also sometimes involved.

In both necrosis and dermatitis the constant factor is general avascularity of the affected area and this influences the surgical approach in two ways:

1. Unless the area is excised deeply beyond the damaged zone, the resulting granulations tend to be poor and the chances of a free skin graft taking either at the time of excision or subsequently are poor.

2. The suture holding properties of therapy-damaged skin are bad and the tissues are slow to heal.

Which tissues have borne the brunt of the damage will depend on whether the skin or deeper structures were the primary target of the radiotherapy and this must be assessed before deciding on the type of repair. The mobility of the skin is a good clinical indicator of whether the deeper structures are involved.

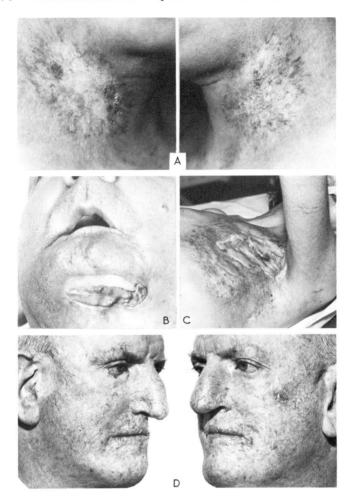

Fig. 6.6 Examples of radionecrosis and radiodermatitis.

A   Radiodermatitis of neck following radiotherapy for thyrotoxicosis.
B   Radionecrosis of chin, floor of mouth, and mandible with fistula, following
     irradiation of squamous carcinoma of floor of mouth. The tube pedicle raised for
     repair of the ulcer is shown in Figure 4.8A.
C   Radionecrosis of chest wall resulting from radiotherapy following radical mastec-
     tomy for carcinoma, showing central deep ulceration with exposure of ribs, and
     surrounding radiodermatitis.
D   Radiodermatitis following radiotherapy for acne vulgaris. Free skin grafts of right
     lower eyelid and right pre-auricular region are present and since this record was
     made further rodent ulcers have been removed as they appeared.

A further example of radiodermatitis is shown in Figure 4.43A following radiotherapy
for sycosis barbae.

If skin alone is damaged, excision and replacement with a split-skin graft or whole skin graft is usually satisfactory. If, on the other hand, an ulcer is present, it may be assumed that deeper tissues are grossly involved. In such a situation, a blood carrying flap will be needed and excision of the ulcer should be as radical as is technically feasible deeply, clearing therapy-damaged skin at the margins. If bone is involved a sequestrectomy may be done simultaneously. Unfortunately where sequestrectomy is needed the margins of necrosis are difficult to define and this is especially true of the mandible which is often the bone involved.

Before any ulcer is treated a biopsy must be considered to exlude malignancy since this will naturally influence the extent and depth of excision. In this connection it is worth remembering that a malignant ulcer developing in therapy-damaged skin is seldom clinically typical and recurrences of skin tumours following radiotherapy are very liable to masquerade as radionecrosis until biopsy reveals the true state of affairs. When a postirradiation tumour recurrence is being excised the entire area of therapy change should be regarded as suspect even although the visible recurrence is only a small segment of this for the area of therapy change represents the surface extent of the original tumour.

INFECTIVE SKIN LOSS

With the advent of the antibiotics skin necrosis from fulminating cellulitis is uncommon but massive skin loss from infection may still occur as a result of necrotising fasciitis. The primary pathological state is in the superficial fascia where there is a rapidly spreading necrosis. Loss of the overlying skin follows but is secondary, the result of avascular necrosis as its nutrient vessels thrombose.

Treatment consists of wide excision of the involved fascia. The overlying skin, incidentally sacrificed in the fascial excision, may still be healthy if excision has been timely and radical. When this is so it may be possible, using the Gibson Ross (p. 196) dermatome, to cut a split-skin graft from the resected tissue and store it, refrigerated, ready to be applied to the defect once the condition is controlled and the bed healthy.

If the skin cannot be salvaged in this way split-skin grafting is carried out in the usual way once the raw surface has produced healthy looking granulations free of important pathogens. Whether or not the grafts are left exposed or dressed depends largely on the site of the defect.

With either infection the problem of skin cover arises once the infection has been controlled and in both instances two conditions must be satisfied—the granulations must look healthy with evidence of marginal healing, and the bacterial flora must be innocuous. Probably stamp grafts closely placed are the appropriate type of repair; they are certainly the safest.

POSTSURGICAL SKIN LOSS

A postsurgical skin defect may arise as a result of excision of a tumour of skin itself or one involving skin secondarily, as in carcinoma of breast. Skin grafting has also been used in the treatment of certain anal conditions.

NEOPLASIA OF SKIN

It is essential in treating malignant skin tumours that the surgeon should separate, in his mind at least, the excision of the tumour and the repair of the defect so that the tumour will be treated according to its nature and extent witout regard to possible problems of repair.

The head and neck apart, the policy of skin replacement following excision of a malignant tumour of skin is a straightforward one. The cosmetic aspect is of minor significance as a factor in deciding type of repair and the split-skin graft applied immediately after excision is the usual method employed. The free skin graft has the advantages in this field of being technically easier and of not obscuring the field when recurrence is being watched for.

One of the few situations which might call for the primary use of a flap would be one where excision leaves a surface which cannot take a free skin graft, for example cortical bone or tendon. The advantages of flap cover must then be weighed against the degree of certainty of adequate excision.

The pros and cons of immediate flap repair arise with greater urgency in neoplasia of head and neck and will be considered in detail then but much of the argument applies to the problem elsewhere in the body. In practice the flap has a very minor role in providing immediate skin cover following excision of a malignant skin tumour.

NEOPLASIA OF THE HEAD AND NECK

This subject is a vast one and will be discussed only as it affects the surgical procedure. As in other fields of surgery pathology should govern practice. So many malignant neoplasms of head and neck are 'local conditions' that adequacy of excision becomes of paramount importance and thoughts of subsequent repair should not influence excision if this will in any way contravene pathological considerations. Many lesions are of course small enough to be excised and the defect closed by direct suture. The problem really arises when the defect is large enough to require more formal repair. Such defects require either a free skin graft or a flap and if a flap is used the type most often appropriate is a local flap.

Skin tumours occur in two ways on the face—as single lesions in the midst of clinically normal skin and as multiple lesions in sun-damaged skin. The single lesion tends to be well-defined and clinically typical; the multifocal lesion has ill-defined margins and is often atypical. The management of the two types is quite different as regards repair.

In the management of the multifocal lesion with actinic damaged skin all around there is little place for the local flap. The skin of any local flap will itself almost certainly be showing pathological changes similar in nature to those of the excised area which, though they may be less advanced, can nonetheless be expected to progress to full-blown neoplasia in a percentage of cases. Such skin in any case is often atrophic and quite unsuited for use as a flap. The free skin graft is to be preferred as a general rule.

In the single lesion the decision is less clear cut. Often the flap would give a much better cosmetic result and solely on those grounds would be preferable. The free skin graft on the other hand, with the exception of the postauricular whole skin graft around eye and nose, gives a relatively poor cosmetic result. Despite this its merit on pathological grounds is unassailable for its use allows inspection of the operative field for any recurrence and permits early biopsy of any area which is remotely suspicious. Recurrence deep to a flap is apt to be disastrously large before its presence is sufficiently evident clinically to tempt the surgeon to interfere with his flap. Certainly clearance in depth is essential when the use of a flap is contemplated.

Where the slightest doubt of clearance exists, particularly in depth, the proper policy is generally to repair excisional defects where at all possible with free skin grafts, including where necessary the wearing of prostheses. When the area has been watched for 9 to 18 months according to the local and pathological circumstances until any recurrence is likely to have appeared, a reassessment can be made and the definitive repair proceeded with if this is felt desirable. A permanent prosthesis sometimes gives the best result and if so may be considered as the definitive 'repair' (Fig. 6.7).

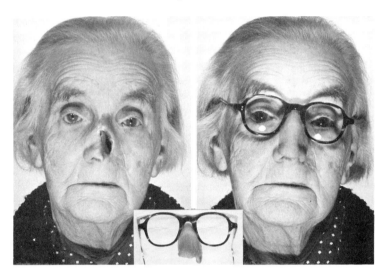

Fig. 6.7 Acrylic prosthesis as permanent 'repair' or nasal defect following excision of a basal cell carcinoma. The age and general condition of the patient were considered to preclude definitive repair with the patient's own tissues.

Further examples of prosthetic repairs are shown in Figures 4.33 and 6.20.

There may of course be overriding circumstances which dictate departure from this principle and examples are:

1. Where a gross salivary fistula will be produced by the excision. This applies expecially to older patients who do not tolerate a fistula well; in such circumstances it is wise to aim at primary definitive repair. In any case such excisions usually involve the full thickness of cheek or lip and marginal recurrence alone need be watched for.

2. Where bare skull will be produced by an excision a rotation flap is needed. Fortunately deep clearance can be more assured here than in most other situations.

3. Where deep clearance is clinically definite but during excision temporomandibular joint or mandible is exposed. Neither is capable of taking a free skin graft and the trismus produced if either is left to granulate before grafting makes a flap necessary.

4. Where it proves impossible to achieve complete excision of a tumour it may be worth while to rotate a flap for skin cover so that further radiotherapy can be given.

Excluding the free skin graft, and there are no special points to distinguish graft usage in the head and neck from elsewhere except the technical problems arising from the need of the patient to breathe and eat, the types of repair can best be illustrated by reference to the various parts of the head and neck involved.

The lips

The type of repair depends on whether a full-thickness defect results from the excision requiring lining to be transferred with the flap employed.

Full thickness defects

V-excision and direct closure (Fig. 6.8). Up to one-third of either lip can be excised and directly closed without unduly constricting the

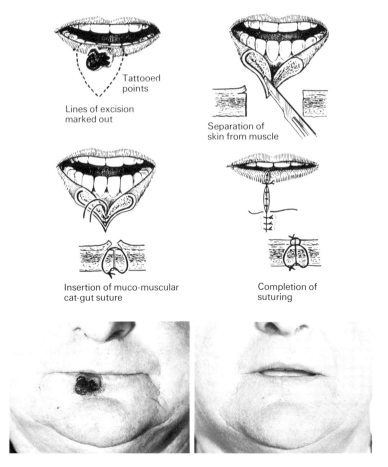

Fig 6.8 Squamous carcinoma of lower lip treated by V-excision with direct suture showing the two-layer method of suture which is routinely used in repairing the full thickness of the lip.

mouth. Suturing, as with all lip repairs, is in two layers. Undermining of the skin for 3 mm or so defines the mucomuscular layers which are united with vertical mucomuscular mattress catgut sutures. These sutures take the strain of the repair and allow the skin edges to be closed without tension or tendency to invert. It is usual in cleft lips to incorporate a Z-plasty of the red margin to give a smoother margin to the lip but in cancer surgery it is preferable to use straight suture for this leaves a single line only to be watched for recurrence.

Many of these patients show diffuse premalignant change of the exposed area of the whole length of red margin and this can be treated by excising the affected strip, advancing the mucosa inside the mouth round to meet the skin—the 'lip shave' (Fig. 6.9). There is no need to mobilise the mucosa prior to advancement and in fact mobilisation is liable to lead to marginal necrosis of the advanced mucosa. When the main lesion is regarded either as premalignant or not yet invasive the lip shave can replace the V-excision and it can also be used to remove the premalignant red margin after the V-excision has removed the area of frank clinical carcinoma.

The V-lip-switch flap. This consists of the transfer of a full-thickness flap, pedicled on the labial vessels, from one lip to fill a correspondingly shaped defect of the other lip (Fig. 6.10). The flap is usually V-shaped; various eponyms are applied to the several varieties. It is a useful repair when the central one-third to a half of a lip has been removed and in such a case the lips are attached to each other by the narrow pedicle until it can safely be divided two weeks later. Where a V has been excised near the angle (Fig. 6.11) the switched flap can also be used and the pedicle becomes then the new angle of mouth.

Fan flap. When more than half of a lip or a rectangular segment has been excised, the V-lip-switch flap is less effective and a flap corresponding in shape to the defect must be used. Since neoplasms of the lower lip are much more common it is the defect of the lower lip which usually calls for repair.

A fan-shaped flap based on the labial vessels of the normal lip and of depth corresponding to the defect is constructed and rotated to fill the defect. The secondary defect is closed by taking up the slack present on the cheek. It is fortunate that most repairs are carried out in the older age group where adequate slack in the cheek is usually available.

The flap can be rotated until flap red margin meets lip red margin (Fig. 6.12) but this reduces the size of the mouth considerably. An alternative method which is particularly useful in repairs following extensive lip resections is to suture the skin and mucosa of the flap

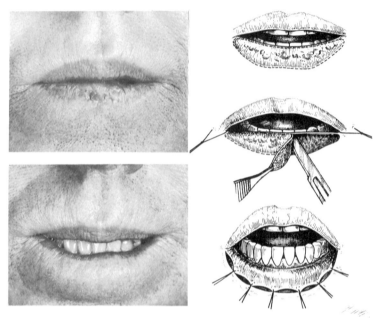

Excision of red margin and mucosal advancement —"lip-shave"

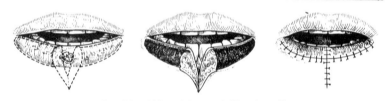

Combined V-excision and "lip-shave"

Fig. 6.9 Excision of premalignant margin of lower lip and repair by 'lip-shave'. As indicated this method of repair can be combined with a V-excision if necessary.

along the line of resection and use it as the red margin (Fig. 6.13). This often leaves a larger mouth. In practice the best method is that in which the flap lies most easily.

It may happen that the angle of mouth has to be opened up secondarily if the orifice is too small. This should if anything be underdone as the opened segment tends to gape in a rather unsightly manner.

Bilateral fan flaps can be used to repair a defect of the entire lower lip (Fig. 6.14). In such a situation skin to mucosal suture must be used to reconstitute the red margin as the alternative method

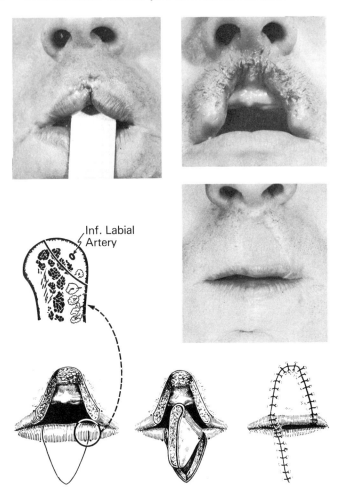

Fig. 6.10 Basal cell carcinoma of central upper lip closed initially by skin-mucosal suture. Definitive repair with a V-flap pedicled on the inferior labial vessels and switched from lower to upper lip.

approximating red margins would make the orifice of the mouth impossibly small.

Skin and muscle defects

The potential source of material for repair depends on the size of the defect. When the defect is of any size the main sources are the forehead and neck. For the upper lip and nasolabial region (Fig. 6.15) flaps of forehead skin pedicled on the temporal vessels are

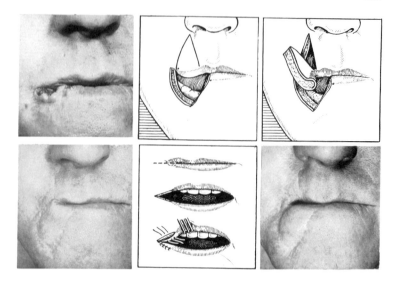

Fig. 6.11 Squamous carcinoma near the angle of the lower lip excised and repaired with a V-flap from the upper lip. Angle of mouth opened subsequently.

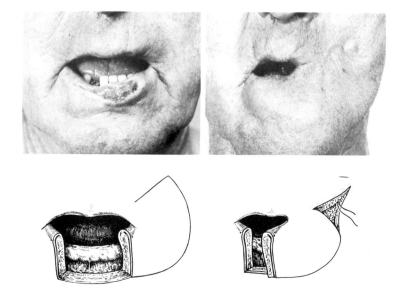

Fig. 6.12 Excision of two-thirds of lower lip for squamous carcinoma and repair with a single fan flap rotating red margin to meet red margin showing the reduction in the size of the mouth which results. The patient refused further surgery to enlarge the aperture of the mouth.

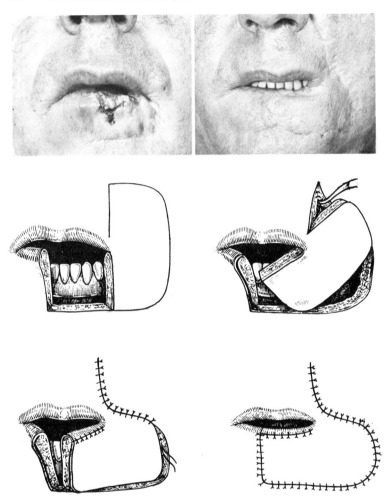

Fig. 6.13 Recurrence of squamous carcinoma of lower lip following radiotherapy excised and repaired by single fan flap with reconstruction of the red margin by advancing mucosa.

usual. Rotation or transposed flaps for the lower lip (Fig. 6.16) are usually taken from the neck either with a secondary free skin graft to the donor site or direct closure if the skin is sufficiently lax.

The nose

For small defects, particularly where there is no loss of lining, the forehead is the usual source of skin. To cover the upper nose and

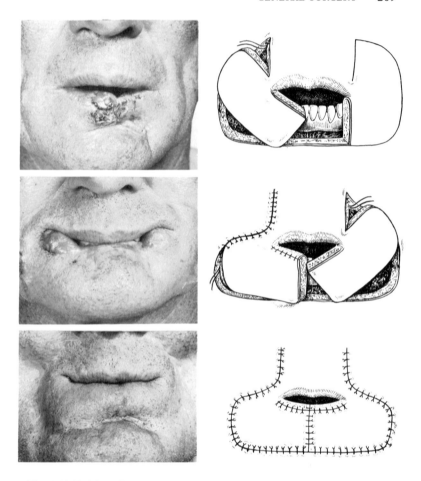

Fig. 6.14 Excision of almost the entire lower lip for squamous carcinoma. Initial closure by skin-mucosal suture and subsequent repair by bilateral fan flaps.

adjoining canthal area a flap based on one set of supra-orbital vessels can be rotated leaving a forehead defect which can usually be closed by direct suture (Fig. 6.17 and 4.34).

The reach of this flap is strictly limited and beyond it the usual complication which arises in considering repair if the defect is of full-thickness is need of lining. The methods of coping with this problem are beyond the scope of this book. If no lining is needed, the forehead bridge pedicle flap based either on the temporal (Fig. 4.33) or supraorbital vessels (Fig. 6.18) is most useful though with a smaller defect a nasolabial flap may be possible.

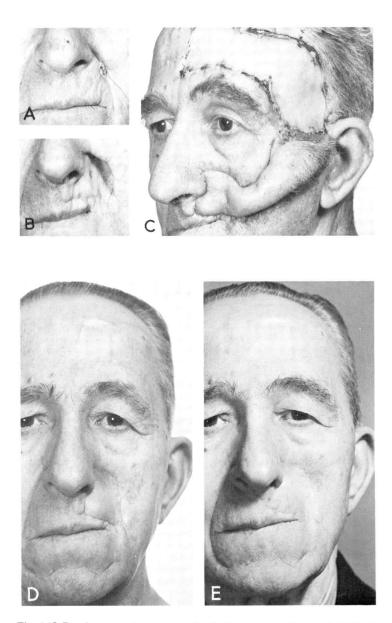

Fig. 6.15 Deeply penetrating morpheic basal cell carcinoma of nasolabial fold (A), excised and repaired primarily with a split-skin graft (B). Definitive repair with temporal bridge pedicle flap (C) after excision of the split-skin graft. Immediate result (D) and final result (E) after scar excisions incorporating Z-plasties.

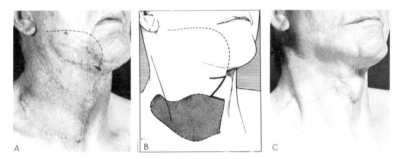

Fig. 6.16 Basal cell carcinoma overlying and invading the body of the mandible, excised and repaired by transposed flap.

A   Extent of excision and delay of flap.
B   Transfer of flap with development of web across the chin and Z-plasty outlined.
C   End result after Z-plasty.

The cheek

The most useful method of repair using local tissues is the inferiorly based rotation flap by which pre-auricular skin is brought forward (Fig. 6.19 and 4.26). The defect posteriorly can usually be closed, but when a free skin graft is needed its relatively inconspicuous position gives a good cosmetic result. The method works best where the lesion is long and narrow or can readily be triangulated.

For the larger defect, skin has usually to be brought from a distance and the deltopectoral flap is in many cases the simplest method (Fig. 4.35).

The ear

Complicated reconstructions of ear following limited excision are described but reasonably good results can be obtained by very simple methods (Fig. 6.20). With a tumour confined to the ear, two courses are open:

1. When the lesion is neither meatal nor peripheral and is small enough to be excised leaving enough ear to make reconstruction worth while, a simple V-shaped full-thickness excision with the apex towards the meatus and the limbs of the V of equal length should be used giving adequate tumour clearance. Closure of the defect by suturing the limbs of the V together in the two skin layers produces some distortion, but in most cases is entirely adequate cosmetically (Fig. 6.20A). When good prosthetic facilities are available an alternative method may be to leave the defect fully displayed by suturing the skin on the two sides of the ear together. The residual ear can be made the basis of a partial prosthesis (Fig. 6.20B).

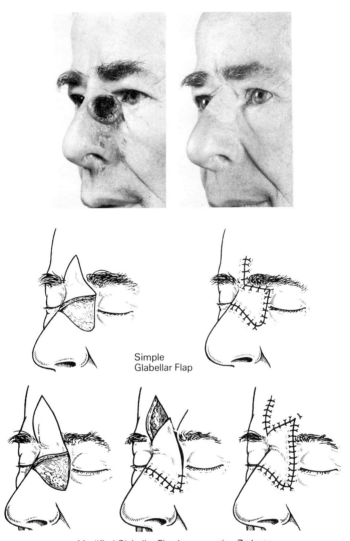

Simple
Glabellar Flap

Modified Glabellar Flap incorporating Z-plasty

Fig. 6.17 Very extensive kerato-acanthoma, confirmed by clinical behaviour and biopsy, excised and repaired by simple glabellar flap. A modification is also shown which is useful when there is difficulty in closing the secondary defect of forehead.

2. The peripheral lesion can be dealt with by adequate clearance of the tumour followed by an additional excision of 6 mm of cartilage to allow the skin to be closed directly over it.

There should be no hesitation, however, in excising the ear

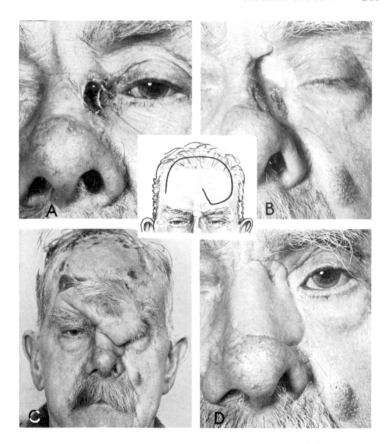

Fig. 6.18 Penetrating basal cell carcinoma of medial canthus and adjoining nose (A), excised and repaired primarily with a split-skin graft (B). After a period of follow-up without recurrence definitive repair by forehead bridge pedicle flap (inset and C). Result following return of bridge segment (D). The patient refused to have further trimming, etc., of the flap.

completely and, if necessary, of removing adjoining skin, etc. A free skin graft does well in this site, making an appropriate incision to correspond to the meatal stump (Fig. 6.20c). The ear is one of the easiest appendages to replace effectively either with a partial or total prosthesis.

CARCINOMA OF BREAST

Radical mastectomy involves removal of a large area of skin and further skin loss may be caused by suturing the wound under tension. This has led to an increasing awareness of the value of the

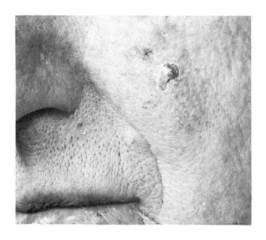

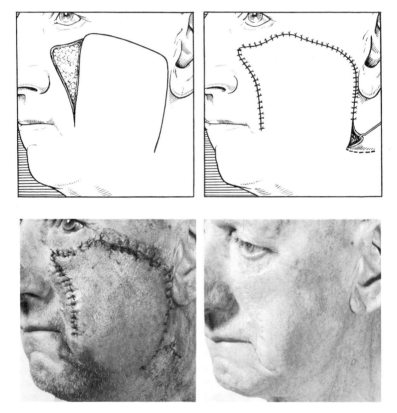

Fig. 6.19 Early invasive squamous carcinoma of cheek arising on a background of actinic damage, excised and repaired by modified rotation flap using the method described in Figure 4.32.

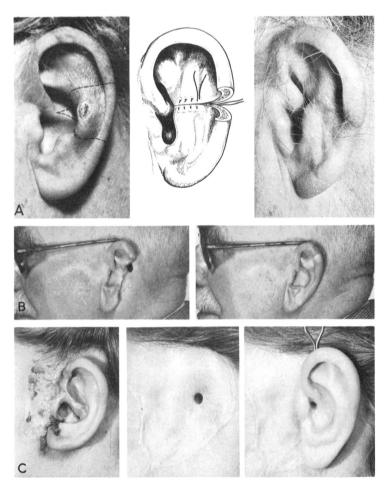

Fig. 6.20 Repairs following excision of neoplasms of ear.

A   V-excision of squamous carcinoma of pinna with direct closure of defect.

B   Acrylic prosthetic replacement following partial excision of helix for squamous carcinoma.

C   Extensive basal cell carcinoma of pre-auricular skin involving the pinna by direct spread, radically excised and repaired by split-skin graft and acrylic prosthesis.

free skin graft following mastectomy. The usual graft used is a thick split-skin graft and the essential point of technique is to ensure close and immobile contact of graft and chest wall. The skin flaps are liable to be mobile and it is unwise to rely on them alone for anchorage. Various methods are described to give added fixation but as simple as any is to make the graft overlap the defect so that it extends on to the flaps. The usual anchoring suture with a bite through intercostal muscle or rib periosteum will fix both graft and flap to the chest wall.

By leaving the sutures long as usual a tie-over bolus dressing can be used to give the necessary local immobility. The flaps can be independently drained or treated by continuous suction as preferred; the graft still remains a separate entity fixed to the chest wall.

An alternative method which can be used to provide cover when breast skin has been excised is the latissimus dorsi myocutaneous flap (p. 173). This flap is particularly valuable if the question of prosthetic replacement of the resected breast tissue is being considered. Prosthetic replacement following mastectomy is being viewed more and more as a possibility and the need for flap rather than graft replacement of resected breast skin is increasing in consequence.

SURGERY OF THE ANUS AND VULVA

In the treatment of fistula-in-ano, anal fissure and anal stenosis it is usual practice to leave at the end of the surgical procedure a widely open, saucerised or flat, raw area to epithelialise slowly from its margins. By grafting this area considerable reduction in healing time can be achieved. Indeed the methods used to cure the pathological condition and prevent its recurrence, namely the eradication of fistulous tracks, the prevention of pocketing by wide skin excision, and the conversion of the wound into a single, widely open cavity, are the very points one would stress in laying down principles of successful grafting under such conditions.

The natural resistance of the perineum to its normal flora would appear to extend to skin grafts and infection is seldom a problem given good contact between graft and recipient site and no dead space full of haematoma or tissue fluid to provide a culture medium. As haematoma is the most likely cause of graft loss, adequacy of haemostasis becomes the deciding factor in whether the graft can safely be applied immediately on concluding the anal surgery or whether it is better applied as a secondary prodecure two days later. The superficial, flat surface can readily be grafted immediately but the deeper cavity left after the treatment of an anorectal fistula where haemostasis is more difficult is probably better left for secondary grafting. When secondary grafting is being used the wound can be packed for the two days and then gently cleared of clot to receive the graft. With either method massive catgut ligatures should be avoided.

The actual method of applying the graft does not differ from elsewhere; a split-skin graft overlapping the margin of the raw surface is used with the usual tie-over dressing. A thin split-skin graft is preferable because of its better taking properties. The secondary contraction of such a graft is of no moment and such contraction as does occur can be turned to advantage in reducing the depth of the grafted cavity.

After the first dressing on the fourth to fifth day all dressings are discarded and the bowel can safely be opened if the area is gently and carefully cleaned afterwards. The use of a skin graft need not influence the administration of intestinal antibiotics as a cover during surgery of the anal condition.

It is a fortunate coincidence that the surgical steps essential for good graft take should be those necessary to eliminate the particular pathological condition for it means that partial or even complete failure of the graft to take is not an irreparable disaster; local treatment can, if necessary, proceed as though a graft had never been used.

In the occasional neoplasm of the anal and peri-anal skin a similar approach can be used successfully (Fig. 6.21) though the poorly vascular fat of the ischiorectal fossa is exposed by tumour excision is not the best bed for a graft and take is hazardous on this account alone. An alternative to early grafting is to await granulations and

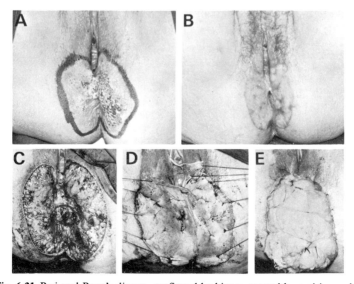

Fig. 6.21 Peri-anal Paget's disease, confirmed by biopsy, treated by excision and grafting. (A) shows the lesion with the marginal clearance marked out in Bonney's Blue, and (B) the final result. (C) shows the excision, (D) the graft applied, with additional quilting sutures for additional anchorage, and (E) the tie-over dressing.

then graft, either exposed or with dressings, whichever seems appropriate. The difficulty then becomes that of getting the area clean and fit for grafting, a problem which varies with the weight and build of the patient. Probably if anything primary grafting is preferable unless the tumour is grossly infected.

The problem in the vulvar area is rather different and arises from the need to resurface the raw surface left after the radical vulvectomy and bilateral clearance of inguinal lymph nodes with overlying skin

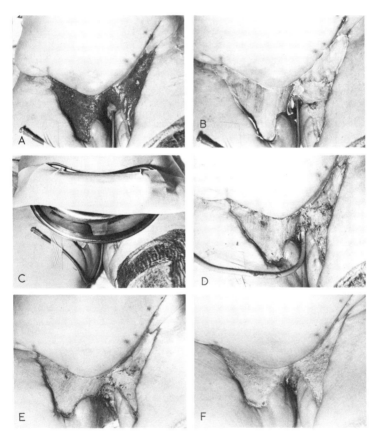

Fig. 6.22 Squamous carcinoma of vulva treated by radical vulvectomy followed by delayed exposed grafting. Fourteen days after vulvectomy the raw surface is granulating satisfactorily (A) and is ready to receive the split-skin graft, cut the previous day and stored overnight. The indwelling catheter is in position. The graft is applied as sheets (B) and is protected by the inverted kidney dish (C). Removal of the kidney dish on the 5th day (D) shows the graft. (E) shows the graft on the 12th day and (F) the final result.

which is the standard surgical treatment of carcinoma of the clitorovulvar region. In this situation primary grafting has had its occasional and very dramatic successes but most surgeons have to report much more frequent failures. It is technically a very difficult region to graft successfully primarily.

A safe and simple alternative is to await granulations and graft secondarily using the exposure method (Fig. 6.22). Once granulations are well established the actual operation merely consists of cutting the skin graft. The skin can then be stored until the patient is awake and co-operative back in bed with Foley catheter in position and legs held slightly abducted with sand-bags. The graft can then be laid on the granulations and protected for five days or so with an inverted kidney dish.

Quite apart from its safety and simplicity this method has the advantage of dividing the procedure into two distinct parts and allows the patient, frequently old and rather frail, to be ambulant during preparation for grafting. Delayed grafting in addition makes for an easier convalescence from the vulvectomy than primary grafting.

Skin flaps in anovulvar defects tend to do badly and they are not recommended. A very effective alternative when the defect is not suitable for grafting is the gracilis myocutaneous flap. The closeness of its pivot point to the ischiopubic ravus makes the flap ideally sited to resurface defects in this area.

7

Orthopaedic surgery

Skin cover in orthopaedic surgery is required because of the need for a sterile field during and after surgery of bone and joint. In acute bony trauma with skin deficiency, skin cover can for practical purposes convert an open into a closed fracture with a corresponding drop in the probability of infection. In the late treatment of trauma adequate skin cover permits an operative approach without fear of wound breakdown and infection. When secondary surgery of nerve or tendon is required good skin cover is equally necessary for similar reasons.

The care of the paraplegic has become a matter for the orthopaedic surgeon and the surgery of decubitus ulceration will be considered in this context. The problem of pressure sores extends to the non-paraplegic but the principles of surgical treatment apply to both types of ulcer and they will be discussed together.

SKIN COVER IN BONY TRAUMA

In civilian life the fractures most commonly associated with skin loss are of the subcutaneous long bones, tibia and less often ulna. The aim of treatment in such an injury is to prevent infection, first by **fixing the fracture** and second by **providing skin cover** to isolate it from the surface.

Provision of skin cover

These combined injuries of skin and skeleton can occur in all degrees of severity from the compound fracture with minimal skin loss up to the extensive degloving associated with a compound fracture and/or a joint injury. It is the injury of the latter type which usually poses the major technical problems.

In the case of the compound fracture with minimal skin loss a 'relaxation' incision is often recommended as a way of achieving skin closure. The idea is to reduce tension by making a 'relaxing' incision at some distance from the wound and in this way allow safe suture, the secondary defect being split-skin grafted. The method sounds simple and safe enough, but it is important to appreciate that such a 'relaxing' incision really creates a bipedicled strap flap. It is a well-recognised fact that even in optimal circumstances the bipedicled strap flap is basically an unsafe procedure and often results in a large slough. Used in a mixed skin and skeletal injury it is even more hazardous for soft tissue damage and degloving have so often added their quota to the local devitalisation of skin. The presence of degloving should in fact be a virtual contra-indication and even in the absence of degloving its use must always be assessed with the greatest of care. The incision itself should run in the long axis of the limb; it should be placed at a considerable distance from the wound and undermining of the skin should be avoided if at all possible. The method is likely to be of most use when there has been no significant skin loss and closure is difficult because of the local swelling of the limb from oedema and haemorrhage.

The compound fracture with skin loss of greater or lesser degree is a very different proposition and a much more difficult problem. Before the management of these more severe injuries is discussed, however, it is important to understand the underlying principles, for the detailed handling of a patient is at all times the expression in practical terms of these principles.

The first concerns the crucial role of the periosteum in relation to skin cover. *Cortical bone covered with periosteum can be expected to take a split-skin graft; cortical bone denuded of periosteum cannot be expected to take a split-skin graft*. It follows that while the surgeon has to accept those therapeutic problems posed by the cortical bone denuded by the injury he should not add to the bare bone and consequent problems by his subsequent activities.

The second concerns possible types of skin cover and in particular their limitations in this context. Four methods are available—**skin flap, free skin graft, muscle or myocutaneous flap** and **free flap** using microvascular anastomotic techniques. Combinations of these methods are also possible.

Skin flaps. It can be stated straightaway that local flaps, rotation or transposed, have no place in acute injuries of this sort. The possible flap would therefore most probably be a direct one, in the upper limb from the trunk, in the lower limb from the uninjured limb as a cross-leg flap. Restrictions on the use of flaps in such circumstances are considerable. No preliminary delay is possible and the length-breadth ratio becomes much more crucial with something like a one to two ratio of length to breadth necessary for safety. Even then such a flap would be hazardous used by someone lacking previous experience of flap transfers. Flaps are not feasible even as elective procedures in older patients because of peripheral vascular problems in the ageing limb and problems of joint stiffness. These considerations apply with redoubled force in emergency situations especially in the lower limb where the problem really arises.

This means that in a lower limb injury a cross-leg flap can be contemplated only by the experienced operator in the young patient with unimpaired peripheral circulation and joints capable of tolerating the necessary immobilisation. The presence of degloving with skin necrosis much beyond the width of the subcutaneous border of the tibia and beyond its length completely rules it out. The more localised the skin loss the more feasible is it likely to be and then to accommodate a flap broad enough to have a 1:2 length-breadth ratio the original defect may have to be enlarged by excising normal skin adjoining it. The fracture must be simultaneously stabilised, if need be by plating or intramedullary nailing whichever is appropriate and such a method can only be used if the fracture is seen soon after injury and adequate debridement can be carried out. As can be imagined the number of potentially suitable candidates is extremely small.

Free skin graft. Even with alternatives available it remains true that split-skin grafting should be used if the raw surface permits it. In deciding which surfaces to graft the role of the periosteum as a key structure has constantly to be borne in mind. Excision of avascular soft tissue, conservation of periosteum, closure of open joint by suture of the capsule when possible, fixation of the fracture—all these combine to give a graft the best possible chance to take. The split-skin graft has the great virtue on occasion of stabilising a clinical situation at minimal cost to the patient. It permits the surgeon a breathing space and even if it is undesirable as definitive cover a graft can always be replaced at leisure once the patient's condition has become stable.

The split-skin graft can also of course be used in conjunction with other techniques. A muscle flap, for example, may be needed to cover the bare bone component of a composite injury involving skin and bone but a split-skin graft can still be applied all around as well as providing the skin cover over the muscle.

Muscle and myocutaneous flaps. This method of providing cover has been applied with greatest effect in defects of the knee and anterior tibia. The medial head of gastrocnemius is able to cover the upper third of the tibia and the medial aspect of the knee joint; the middle third requires the transfer of soleus, reinforced if need be by flexor digitorum longus.

If the appropriate muscle is available its transfer should be regarded as probably the most suitable method of covering bare bone and any plates or screws. Whether transfer of the overlying skin with the muscle as a myocutaneous flap is preferable to transfer of the muscle alone followed by grafting is debatable.

Free flaps. This highly sophisticated method in which an axial pattern flap is transferred as a free flap with anastomosis of its arteriovenous system to vessels in the recipient site has been used with good effect in this type of problem, particularly when the lower tibia is exposed. This area is one not readily covered by any of the other methods.

It is outwith the scope of this book to discuss the technical details of free flap transfers but the patient with an extensive, mixed injury below the knee should certainly have the benefit of at least the opinion of someone familiar with microsurgical techniques and conversant with their applications. There is no doubt that there are patients whose limbs have been saved by their timely use, particularly where the composite transfers of skin and bone, which employ the same techniques of microvascular anastomosis, have been successfully carried out.

Fixation of the fracture

The precise mode of bony fixation is really a matter for the orthopaedic surgeon and will depend at least partly on how unstable the fracture is. In the unstable, mobile fracture associated with degloving, however, it is being increasingly recognised that internal fixation, using the biologically inert metals now available, far from being contraindicated, is frequently very necessary. Fixation may take the form of plate and screws, or screws alone if the fracture is oblique. Even the intramedullary nail has been advocated though the fact that it brings the whole medullary cavity into direct continuity with the fracture and hence the surface may well give the surgeon pause. A further method uses Hoffman's external fixator. In this technique, as applied to the tibia, three transfixion pins are passed through each end of the bone and an external fixation device is used to maintain the bone ends in a fixed position which stabilises the fracture. The method, though effective in the hands of the experienced user, is very elaborate. It would preclude the transfer of a cross-leg flap and might create problems even with a muscle transfer.

Whatever form of fixation, internal or external, is used, however, it is failure to fix the fracture adequately which leads to infection in such a situation—movement and not metal is responsible.

It has already been stressed in relation to skin cover how important is the integrity of the periosteum. In the handling of the fracture too it plays a crucial role. Apart from its effectiveness as a barrier to infection much of the blood supply to the superficial cortex derives from it. This explains why avascular necrosis of the superficial cortex and surface sequestration are probably inevitable where bone has been denuded of periosteum by the injury. It is an added reason why nothing. should be done in manipulating and fixing the fracture which might add to the periosteum already damaged or denude more bone. Plates and screws must therefore be applied on top of periosteum even although this may add to the technical difficulty of fixation.

In the arm a direct flap applied primarily is not likely to pose any major technical problems other than those of achieving an adequate length-breadth ratio by the methods already described but in practice the need for a primary flap in a compound fracture of forearm must rarely arise. The muscular cover of the arm bones is normally complete except for a single border of the ulna. With the fracture reduced the reconstitution of the soft tissues should always leave the fracture minimally compound and a split-skin graft might reasonably be expected to take over the entire area.

In the leg the problems are much greater. The tibia has fully one-third of its surface subcutaneous and a fracture is likely to be much more extensively compound quite apart from the fact that associated skin damage tends to be much more widespread and severe. The limited place of the cross-leg flap has already been stressed but once debrided the raw surface, with the exception of any bone already bare, should be capable of taking a graft. To prepare the surface all non-viable skin is excised along with damaged muscle and any periosteum which is already stripped. Intact periosteum, even if damaged, should not be removed for intact periosteum leaves the possibility of graft take, while periosteum removed leaves only the certainty of graft failure.

With the bone and joint injury reduced, the fracture fixed and the joint capsule if necessary closed by suture, the wound is debrided as described in preparation for grafting.

The split-skin graft is then applied to the entire area as it would be if the injury was a simple degloving injury (see p. 194) recognising of course that it will almost certainly fail over the areas of bare cortical bone. The graft can reasonably be expected to take over a joint closed as described or even slightly open and it may well bridge the fracture if it is well reduced and fixed though in actual practice the site of the skin loss does not invariably coincide with the fracture site. When the two do coincide however it is the presence of bare bone rather than the fracture which will determine take if fixation is good.

At the first dressing 7 to 10 days later the full extent of the skin loss can be assessed accurately and any residual necrotic skin, fat and muscle excised. The general aim then becomes to prepare the area left uncovered to receive skin and as each part granulates to cover it with split-skin. Any internal fixation of the fracture should be left in place, even if it is quite exposed, until the fracture is at least 'sticky'. Where bone is bare a local surface sequestrum will form and granulations can only be expected when it has separated. It is not advisable to excise such dead bone as soon as it is recognised to be dead. Excision at this point is likely to damage the blood supply of the bone which is left and a fresh sequestrum will form. Spontaneous separation should generally be awaited. Sequestrectomy should be carried out reluctantly and only when a good line of demarcation has formed. Time may actually be saved in the long run by waiting for spontaneous separation for granulations will already be present and ready to be grafted when the sequestrum is lifted off.

When skin loss is only recognised late the principles to be followed in providing skin cover are exactly those described above from the time of the first dressing unless the area and other circumstances fit the criteria laid down for the use of a cross-leg flap.

This approach accepting as it does that the split-skin graft rather than the flap is generally going to provide immediate skin cover means that the surgeon may be faced with the subsequent need to replace unstable scar or skin graft with a flap. Subsequent replacement, however, can be carried out in circumstances much more satisfactory than those attending the original injury. Flaps can be properly planned and carefully delayed. In any case there should be no rush to replace graft by flap; the graft supported for a long period with elastic bandaging and permitted time to settle in often becomes stable to a quite unexpected degree. The eventual number of flaps needed will be a mere fraction of the original estimate. Unfortunately the graft most prone to be chronically unstable is the very one where a flap is ruled out because of an ageing limb with poor vascularity and here a regime of elastic bandaging may be needed indefinitely.

Another late problem of mixed skin and bony damage may result from the fact that a secondary orthopaedic procedure, e.g. bone grafting, cannot be carried out through a scarred or even free skin grafted area, especially if the bone is normally subcutaneous, and for that reason alone such scarring may require replacement with a skin or muscle flap. Alternatively, and the possibility should be explored before a flap is used at all the orthopaedic surgeon may be able to use a different surgical approach which avoids the grafted area altogether. When a flap is used in preparation for bone grafting in non-union an incidental benefit to the relatively avascular bone ends is the fresh blood supply which comes with the flap. It is not unknown for the fracture with delayed or seemingly established non-union to unite after the provision of flap cover before there is time to carry out the bone graft which the flap was intended to permit.

OSTEITIS AND INFECTED FRACTURES

In the case of both osteitis and the infected fracture the bone usually involved is the tibia and the problem is either the replacement of unstable scarring from chronic osteomyelitis or the provision of good skin to give the orthopaedic surgeon reasonable material for skin closure when he is exploring the underlying bone or carrying out a sequestrectomy. The actual area of skin replacement and its exact form, whether by skin flap, muscle flap plus split-skin graft or myocutaneous flap, will depend on the local circumstances but it should be generous and planned with enough reserve to cope with the minor infection which may arise from the bone. Precisely when the bone should be tackled in relation to the timing of the flap transfer is a matter for discussion with the orthopaedic surgeon, but in general operation on the diseased bone should be undertaken only if the treated bone can be immediately and completely covered by the flap.

TENDON AND NERVE INJURY

When a nerve or tendon is injured in association with extensive loss of skin it is necessary to provide a covering of subcutaneous tissue as well as skin to form a satisfactory bed prior to any operation of the nerve or tendon itself and a flap must be used as cover. The flap may be transferred as a primary procedure in favourable conditions; alternatively it may be used secondarily once primary healing has been achieved by a split-skin graft.

The methods already described for use in problems involving both skin and bone are equally applicable to this clinical situation.

Occasionally when surgery of bone, joint or tendon is required the skin overlying has to be replaced because disease or previous injury has made it unsuitable. A flap is then usually required (Fig. 7.1).

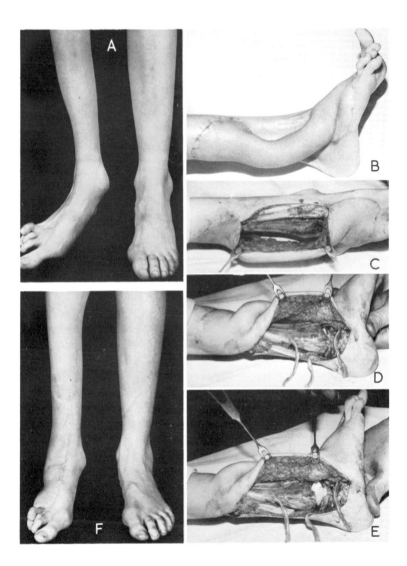

Fig. 7.1 The use of a tube pedicle to replace skin affected by focal scleroderma so that surgery of tendon and joint might be carried out.

A shows the eversion of foot resulting from the focal scleroderma and requiring lengthening of tendons and divisions of the lateral ligaments of ankle joint to permit the foot to take up a normal position. B shows a double attachment of the abdominal tube pedicle with central 'slack' ready to be taken up when the eversion is corrected. C shows the flap untubed and the intervening sclerodermatous skin excised.
D shows the tendons and ligaments divided and E the eversion corrected prior to resuture of the tendons in a lengthened position. F shows the end result with the flap spread and the eversion of the foot corrected.

PRESSURE SORES

Pressure sores occur in bedridden and in paraplegic patients. In both the pathological processes are essentially similar and the cause is pressure sufficiently severe and sustained to produce ischaemic necrosis of the skin. The ulcers develop in areas where pressure is borne and where the pad of subcutaneous tissue is scanty.

THE NON-PARAPLEGIC PRESSURE SORE

Usual sites are the sacral area and heel, occasionally the iliac crest. The cause of the sore, i.e. the factor producing the immobility, must always be treated before considering active surgery of the ulcer; the patient must be capable of keeping off the pressure point.

Local treatment is aimed at getting the ulcer fit for split-skin grafting. When the time comes to apply the graft the problem is usually a technical one of immobilisation and the ingenuity of the surgeon may be taxed to get immobility for the four days or so necessary for graft take. Where all other methods have failed, success has sometimes been achieved by applying closely set thin split-skin stamps without any dressings and merely protected against being rubbed off, the patient being kept on the surface opposite the sore.

If, despite local measures, the ulcer becomes static in size, more heroic measures may be contemplated though the local condition has all too often to be subordinated to the general state of the patient. This is particularly true in sores of the heel where, in theory, the alternative to a split-skin graft would be a cross-leg flap, an alternative quite out of the question in the aged patient. For the sacral area and ilium the alternative to the split-skin graft is usually a rotation or transposed flap, the practice of which will be discussed in relation to the paraplegic.

THE PARAPLEGIC PRESSURE SORE

The areas particularly liable to ulcerate lie over the pressure-bearing bony prominences and in the paraplegic the ulcers tend to have much more of an 'iceberg' quality with extensive undermining and osteitis of the underlying bone or even pyoarthrosis in severe cases. Treatment consists of covering of the completely excised ulcer with a movable pad of healthy skin and subcutaneous tissue and simultaneous elimination of any underlying bony prominence which could act as a focal pressure point. This latter procedure is essential as such prominences left untouched reproduce the mechanical pressure which caused the original ulcer.

During the acute phase of the spinal injury, the common sites are over the sacrum and femoral trochanter; after recovery, prolonged sitting in a wheelchair makes the ischial area the most frequent site. Sacral ulcers tend to be large and flat with minimal undermining; ulcers of the trochanter and ischium usually have a small opening leading into a large slough-lined cavity into the base of which the bony prominence projects.

Healing of the anaesthetic tissues of the paraplegic is poor and with the slightest provocation the wound will fail to heal following surgery. Tension of flaps must be avoided, haemostasis must be even more meticulous than usual, cavities and dead space must be positively eliminated—failure in any one means failure as a whole. When the state of the ulcer permits a preliminary split-skin graft is worth using, for although useless as a definitive procedure it enables the subsequent surgery to be done in a clean surgical field. If skin loss is minimal, excision and direct closure may suffice, but in most cases a rotation or transposed flap is needed. It is seldom possible to avoid grafting the secondary defect but the graft need not necessarily be applied at the actual time of flap transfer. Indeed leaving the secondary defect ungrafted (Fig. 7.3) is a useful way to ensure that a large area is available through which any haematoma can drain instead of collecting under the flap to cause tension, infection and necrosis. The graft can readily be applied 7 to 10 days later.

When multiple sores are present the planning of the several flaps required must be co-ordinated carefully so that the strictly limited areas of available skin are used to the best advantage.

Sacral ulcers

The appropriate type of flap depends on the shape of the ulcer. Frequently suitable is the bilateral rotation flap of buttock skin based on the inferior gluteal fold (Fig. 7.2) and this double flap is especially useful in the sacral pressure sore in the non-paraplegic patient. If the shape and extent of the ulcer make this flap unsuitable, alternatives are the transposed or rotation flap based on the lumbar region (Fig. 7.4), or as a last resort, a tube pedicle. This latter procedure has many technical difficulties and should not be lightly undertaken.

Trochanteric ulcers

Initially, the main cavity of the ulcer is the trochanteric bursa and, if this alone is involved, permanent closure may be achieved without

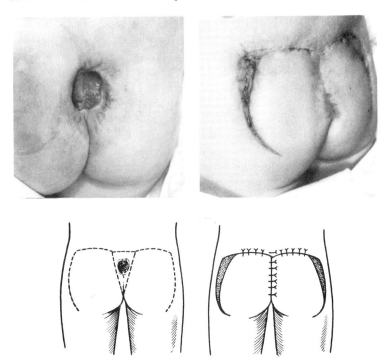

Fig. 7.2 A sacral pressure sore in a non-paraplegic repaired with bilateral rotation—transposed flaps of buttock skin.

interfering with the bone. Frequently, however, the trochanter and neck of femur project into the cavity and excision of trochanter and appropriate cortex of the shaft is then required to let the soft tissues collapse and obliterate the cavity. In the most severe instances a pyoarthrosis of the hip joint develops and once present, this complication is virtually impossible to eradicate without amputation. It is probably wise in such circumstances to concentrate on improving the patient's general condition as much as possible and accept the permanency of the pyoarthrosis.

The ulcer is so undermined in most cases that free skin grafting is seldom practicable. Cover by a local flap is necessary. When this is a skin flap a transposed flap is used (Fig. 7.3); its precise situation and shape will depend on the size and shape of the ulcer, with the proviso always that the secondary defect must be on an area free from subsequent weight-bearing. Added safety can be provided by incorporating the ilio-tibial tract in the flap, in the form of a tensor fasciae latae myocutaneous flap (Fig. 7.7). The donor site is

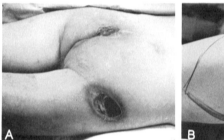
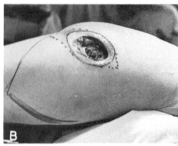

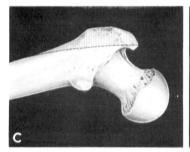
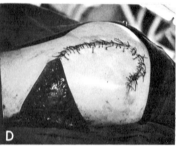

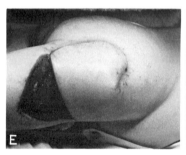
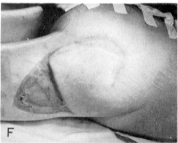

Fig. 7.3 A sacral and a trochanteric ulcer in a paraplegic showing repair of the trochanteric ulcer.

    A   The ulcers.

    B   The trochanteric ulcer with the transposed flap outlined.

    C   The wedge of protruding trochanter excised to eliminate the focal point of pressure.

D and E   The flap transferred, at operation, and 10 days later prior to application of the split-skin graft to the secondary defect.

    F   The end result.

It is not necessary always to graft the secondary defect at the time of the flap transfer. In this patient the secondary defect was grafted 10 days later using the exposed method of grafting.

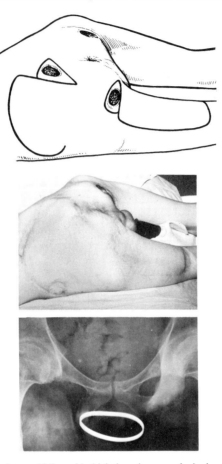

Fig. 7.4 A sacral ulcer and bilateral ischial ulcers in a paraplegic showing repair of the sacral ulcer by a rotation flap of buttock skin and of the left ischial ulcer by a transposed flap of thigh skin. The X-ray shows the extent of the ischiectomy on the left side and the osteitis of the right ischial tuberosity.

adjacent, a 20 cm long flap is likely to be adequate and the secondary defect is not subject to pressure.

Ischial ulcers

The cavity of the ulcer consists of the ischial bursa, but as the condition progresses and extends the ischial tuberosity projects into the cavity and becomes the seat of chronic osteitis. An advance in the treatment of this type of ulcer has been treatment of the ischial tuberosity jointly with the appropriate soft tissue surgery (Fig. 7.4).

Even where the bone is not pathologically involved it is still the main cause of the ulceration.

When planning the appropriate flap the patient should have the hip flexed to imitate the sitting posture to ensure that residual scars do not overlie the tuberosity. The best flap is very broadly based medially along the greater part of the thigh and moved upwards (Fig. 7.5). Its superiority over other possible designs is due to its generous dimensions which on the one hand make it extremely safe

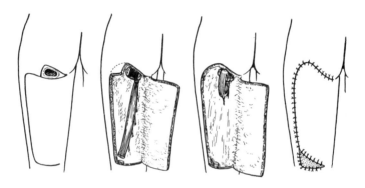

Fig. 7.5 The transposed flap used to repair the defect left following excision of the ischial ulcer and ischiectomy. The cavity left by the ischiectomy is filled by detaching at its lower end and mobilising such hamstring musculature as is available.

and on the other permit further rotation (Fig. 7.6) should the ulcer recur. An added advantage of this flap is that if ischiectomy is made part of the procedure the atrophic remnant of the biceps muscle can be detached at its lower end and mobilised by dividing approximately half of the perforating vessels. The muscle can then be rolled up and tucked into the dead space left by the ischiectomy.

An alternative possibility is the tensor fasciae latae flap. Used for this purpose the flap length needed is rather greater than for the trochanteric ulcer, a flap of 30 cm or even more being required. Where trochanteric and ischial ulcers coexist, the single flap may be able to cover both simultaneously (Fig. 7.7).

The gracilis myocutaneous flap has also been used in ischial ulceration but the muscle in the paraplegic is apt to be insubstantial and the method is not recommended.

Total obliteration of the pressure point by ischiectomy used in conjunction with an appropriate flap for skin cover, appeared to be a promising advance when it was first introduced and early results were certainly excellent. It has been the late results which have

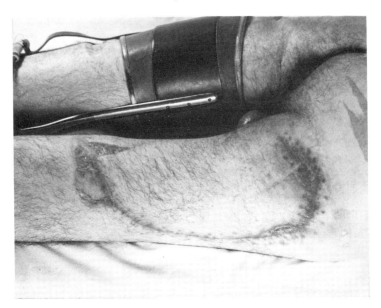

Fig. 7.6 Secondary rotation of a previously used thigh flap to repair recurrent ulceration. The segment of flap beyond the line of the scar of the previous flap was delayed prior to rotation of the flap.

shown up its defects. The major defect as in all procedures in the paraplegic is the tendency to recurrent or fresh ulceration. The difficulty can be stated quite simply—body weight has to be supported somewhere. To state the problem of course does nothing to solve it. So many procedures, particularly where a bony projection is removed, do not really relieve the pressure but merely transfer it to a new area—where the fresh sore develops. This is certainly true of ischiectomy. Following its use ulcers tend to appear on the posterior aspect of the thigh at trochanteric level and also towards the perineum and scrotum. Ulcers in these areas, particularly the perineoscrotal, are most intractable and with flaps already used for ischial sores are very difficult to deal with surgically.

It is probably wiser with the ischial ulcer to compromise and instead of a formal ischiectomy to restrict bony excision to the obvious area of projection.

Certainly it cannot be emphasised too strongly that the procedures which have been described for the various types of decubitus ulceration are only a small facet in the overall care of the paraplegic and must be regarded as merely providing the ulcerated area with a fresh start in the best conditions.

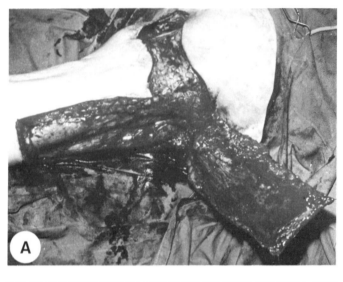

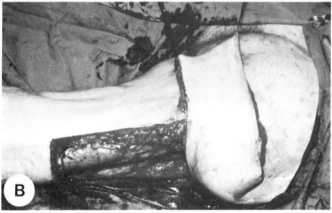

Fig. 7.7 The tensor fasciae latae myocutaneous flap used to provide simultaneous cover for a trochanteric and an ischial pressure sore in a paraplegic patient.
A   The defect and the flap raised.
B   The flap transposed ready for suture.

8

Hand surgery

In surgery of the hand it is essential to avoid the pitfall of seeing the hand in isolation; the patient and his condition must be viewed as one. Before the surgeon embarks on a time-consuming procedure he should give serious thought to whether the end result is going to justify the time spent in obtaining it, with the loss of work and income which the patient will suffer. He must remember that the procedure itself may give rise to disabilities which could outweigh the possible advantages to be derived from it; he must decide whether the patient is intelligent enough to benefit from a complicated reconstruction and co-operate fully during its various stages.

When the alternative exists, a labouring man may well be better off with a partial amputation or a free skin graft of his injured finger than a more elaborate repair which will require immobilisation of one or more fingers or even most of the hand, wrist, elbow and shoulder.

Stiffness of shoulder, arm and hand as a potential complication is especially relevant in the older age group and may be a major consideration in deciding the best procedure.

When different modes of treatment are equally feasible, it is often worth while to explain the problem and its possible solutions in simple terms to the patient so that he may understand what each will entail in time, discomfort and end result. In this way co-operation during the actual procedure is more likely.

HAND INJURIES

In a hand injury the provision of skin cover by direct suture, free skin graft, or flap takes absolute priority. Skin cover alone halts the twin processes of infection and fibrosis which are particularly harmful in the hand. The appropriate method of skin cover depends so much on the type of injury and its extent that an appreciation of the pathological features of the common injury patterns is necessary to an understanding of the principles of treatment.

Hand injuries are of three main types—*cutting and slicing*, *crushing* and *degloving*. As a rule an injury belongs predominantly to one type, but on occasion an injury has the characteristics both of crushing and degloving.

While these three types constitute distinct patterns, injuries of the hand have also been divided from the viewpoint of immediate management into **tidy** and **untidy** injuries, a division which has considerable practical value particularly as it relates to the use of the tourniquet.

In the 'tidy' injury skin damage is clear-cut and the problems of treatment concern more the injury to tendons and nerves. Conditions for accurate and expeditious surgery are therefore essential and a pneumatic tourniquet should be used to provide the necessary bloodless field.

In the 'untidy' injury the main problem concerns viability of tissues. Since the presence or absence of circulation is crucial to such assessment a tourniquet is not used.

CUTTING AND SLICING INJURIES

The extent of a cutting or slicing injury is clear cut and preliminary clinical assessment of damage is straightforward. Tendon and nerve damage are common and must be tested for, but, if one excludes the guillotine amputation which is so often part of the injury, associated bony damage is uncommon. With the exception of the partially sliced off flap, the skin loss is immediately obvious, and even with it the devitalising effect of crushing is not present to add to the difficulty of deciding clinically whether the flap is viable.

It is not proposed to discuss the merits of primary tendon repair; discussion will be concerned rather with the means of providing such skin cover as will permit tendon repair or graft, primarily or secondarily. If exploration or repair of deep structures should be needed the bloodless field created by a pneumatic tourniquet will provide the best conditions for accurate fast surgery.

The method of repair can usually be decided on the basis of the preliminary clinical examination. When there is no loss of skin direct closure with minimal excision of the wound margins should be carried out, and here accurate suturing is as vital as in the face in order to achieve rapid healing with minimal scarring. Skin loss must be made good by free skin graft or flap. Free skin grafts, commonly of split-skin thickness, are generally used except when the raw area includes a structure which will not accept a free skin graft, when the pulp of the finger tip has been lost and replacement requires more bulk than is present in a free skin graft, or when subsequent repair of a deep structure such as tendon is contemplated. In these circumstances flap cover must be provided and the type of flap depends on the site and size of the defect. The possible flaps in the various circumstances will be discussed on page 255.

The guillotine amputation which exposes bone is in many cases best closed by trimming the phalanx until the tissues will close directly over it without tension. Free skin grafts do not do well over such stumps. Failure of the graft over the bone is liable to occur and any scarring adherent to the underlying bone tends to make the graft always vulnerable.

While shortening of a finger to achieve rapid healing may be justified, particularly if only one finger is involved, the approach to the injured thumb is conditioned by the need to maintain length where at all possible. There should be no excessive trimming of a traumatic amputation to get skin cover; a free skin graft or flap should be used as the local circumstances dictate. The overriding need for conservation of finger tissue becomes less with passage towards the ulnar side of the hand.

Finger-tip injuries are liable to present special problems because of the nail and its bed. Their management is discussed on page 243.

Sacrifice of length to get an 'ideal' amputation site is not often justified at the stage of primary treatment. In a single finger injury it may rarely be a reasonable measure, particularly if the loss of length involved is not great, but more often the patient should be given the opportunity to make up his own mind, having used the hand at work, whether or not he wishes secondary shortening carried out.

CRUSHING INJURIES

A crushing injury may vary in severity and extent from the mildest subungual haematoma through the crush injury of fingers with or without bony damage up to the power press injury which leaves a shapeless pulp of devitalised tissue. With severe crushing there is often a 'bursting' laceration. The brunt of the injury is taken by the soft tissues and bones rather than the tendons and nerves. Loss of skin and soft tissue by the actual injury is not a feature but the real loss is often much greater than is at first apparent for disruption of blood vessels and devitalisation of tissues may give rise to quite extensive skin necrosis. This 'hidden' damage may result in unexpectedly severe oedema postoperatively and failure to guard against this oedema can further devitalise the crushed tissues particularly if they have been closed under tension.

Pre-operative appraisal of the situation can be most misleading; only during actual cleansing and surgical exploration of the wound can the injury be accurately assessed. The important points in such an assessment are:

1. To determine what is definitely not viable. The test already described (p. 195) to assess the viability of skin must be rigidly applied here and non-viable soft tissue structures excised quite ruthlessly. This may mean excision of bone, tendon, etc., when a segment of finger as a whole is judged to be non-viable.

2. With the non-viable tissue excised the position is assessed afresh to decide which injured structures are worthy of retention and skin cover. The detailed decisions which this implies must take into account such factors as the relative importance of the fingers and the thumb, the age, intelligence, etc., of the patient, and the extent and severity of the damage.

Much that has been said of closure following guillotine amputation applies to the crushed finger. With the sole exception of the thumb where the conservative approach always applies there are two opposing lines of argument. On the one side the more severe the damage to the individual components of a finger—nerve, tendon, skin, bone, the stronger is the argument for amputation though the finger as a whole may be viable, for the less chance there is of a useful digit resulting. On the other side the greater the damage to other fingers and the rest of the hand the stronger is the argument for retention of the injured digit even in the knowledge that it may be stiff. It is in the crushing injury particularly that a useless finger should always be considered as a potential source of skin. Filleted, it can be used to cover a skin defect of adjoining dorsum or palm avoiding the need for graft or flap.

It is often stated that any lacerations which are present as part of a crushing injury should only be loosely closed with a few tacking sutures because of the tendency to postoperative oedema. In our experience, when no skin has been lost much better results are obtained by suturing such lacerations as accurately as possible with many fine sutures leaving no raw areas between sutures. When this has been followed by absolute immobilisation, preferably with plaster of Paris, and scrupulous postoperative elevation for at least 48 hours oedema has not given rise to any trouble. It seems likely that the oedema which is so feared is the result of failure to follow the latter part of the regime described above.

A relaxing incision, the use of which has been referred to on page 220, can usefully be applied on occasion to the crushed finger when it is proving difficult to close its palmar aspect because of tension. A straight, proximodistal incision through the skin of the dorsum will gape and give enough additional relaxation to allow more ready closure. Here, as in other parts of the limb, undermining must be avoided. The defect caused by the relaxing incision can be split-skin grafted.

Compared with a cutting injury of apparently comparable severity the crushing injury carries a much longer disability period and the results are poorer. The problem of the associated fracture will be considered separately.

DEGLOVING INJURIES

In degloving injuries of the hand, as elsewhere, the important pathological factor is injury to the vascular system. The anatomical characteristics of the palmar skin with its intimate attachment to the the palmar fascia make it less liable to degloving, but when it is degloved the palmar aponeurosis is usually part of the tissue avulsed. Elsewhere the plane is the usual one between superficial and deep fascia.

In the pure degloving injury damage to deeper structures is surprisingly uncommon though it must always be tested for. The important surgical decision is that of viability and skin which is not demonstrably viable (p. 195) must be excised.

The split-skin graft is the usual method of cover and should be used unless tendon, bone or joint is exposed. Even if it is felt that subsequent cover by a flap will be needed the split-skin graft is still the primary cover of choice especially when more than one surface of the hand is involved. When a direct flap is required primarily it should be designed to cover as much of the raw area as possible with its initial attachment.

It is often difficult to estimate the precise skin loss immediately after the injury but over-estimation is less serious than under-estimation. If at the first postoperative dressing skin necrosis is found to be more extensive than was expected and fresh slough is present it should be excised and replaced with a split-skin graft forthwith. In this way healing and mobilisation can be achieved as rapidly as possible.

Degloving of a single digit occurs occasionally and, again with the sole exception of the thumb, amputation is usually advisable. A recommendation which is sometimes made is that a degloved thumb should be 'buried' under the abdominal or chest skin (Fig. 8.1). It should be appreciated however that mere burying of the digit does nothing at all towards providing skin cover. All that can be said is that it buys time but the provision of skin cover has not been advanced in any way. The degloved thumb should instead be inserted into a tubed flap raised on the trunk (Fig. 8.2).

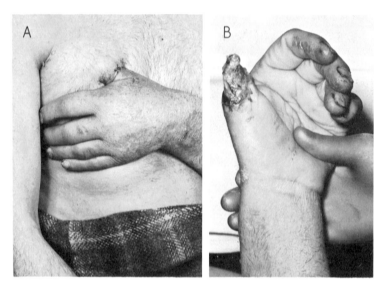

Fig. 8.1 Degloving injury of thumb (A) with loss of distal phalanx treated initially by burying the degloved digit under chest skin. It is apparent (B) that burial of the digit in this fashion has not provided skin cover. Figure 8.2 shows the stages of provision of definitive skin cover.

The use of a tubed flap may be the only way of salvaging the digit though until recently the method did have its limitations and unsatisfactory features. These were due firstly to lack of sensation in the flap which resulted in poor utilisation of the thumb by the patient. Secondly, poor blood supply in the tube resulted in poor tip healing when the flap was separated even after delays, and subsequent inability to withstand cold.

The neurovascular 'island' flap used in this situation has transformed the picture. The hemipulp of a functionally less important finger, usually the ulnar side hemipulp of the ring or middle finger, is raised, pedicled on the digital vessels and nerve, back to their origin in the palm and tunnelled through palm and tube pedicle to a functionally suitable site near the thumb tip. There it is sutured in position (Fig. 8.3). The residual pulp defect is free skin grafted. This brings both nerve and blood supply to the tip with marked improvement in utilisation and vascularity. Sensation is naturally

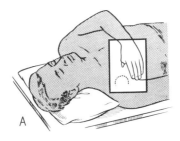

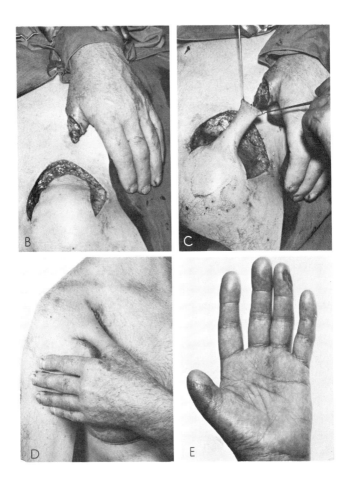

Fig. 8.2 The degloved thumb of Figure 8.1B showing provision of definitive skin cover by pectoral tubed flap, followed by transfer of neurovascular 'island' flap (see Fig. 8.3) to provide sensation. A shows the position of the tubed flap on the chest. B shows the flap raised, and C tube ready to have the thumb inserted. D shows the interval appearance of the tube, and E the final result with the 'island' in position.

projected to the donor finger to begin with and even with use at work over a prolonged period false projection remains in most individuals. Despite this patients adjust remarkably rapidly and do not seem to have any difficulty in use.

The technique is an exacting one and fortunately does not have to be carried out as an emergency. Patients requiring it should probably be referred to a hand surgeon.

FINGER TIP INJURIES

Isolated finger tip injuries of all three types are extremely common and the influence on treatment of the nail and pulp makes separate consideration of the injury necessary.

The pulp with its skin, the phalanx, the nail and its bed, each or all may be damaged in varying degree. The best treatment, by proximal amputation, free skin graft or flap, depends at least partly on the extent of the damage to each constituent. In the extreme case the choice may be clear cut; it is in the mixed injury that difficulty arises. Severe crushing devitalising the nail and phalanx while the pulp is still viable is best treated by amputating the damaged

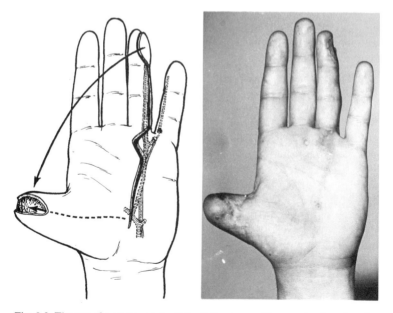

Fig. 8.3 The use of a neurovascular 'island' flap to provide sensation in a thumb resurfaced with a pectoral tubed flap.

segment and closing the defect with a flap of pulp skin. For the slicing injury which removes either pulp skin or distal nail without significantly damaging pulp or phalanx, the obvious measure is a free skin graft. The majority of injuries which lie between these extremes, with loss of pulp and sometimes of bone, are capable of being treated by flap, free skin graft or proximal amputation. The more bone is exposed the less suitable is the site for a free skin graft for the reasons already given (p. 238). The finger tip is one of the very few sites where a whole skin graft has been successfully used in primary trauma, but it has no real advantage over a thick split-skin graft. The all-important need in grafting is for good take; the scar adherent to bone which tends to follow partial take gives a poor result. The common cause of graft failure in this situation is haematoma and in fact haemostasis in a finger tip injury is not always easy to achieve. There is much to be said for postponing the application of the graft for 24 hours to ensure that haemostasis is complete. It is not even essential to suture the graft in position with a tie-over dressing in such circumstances. 'Micropore' tape can be used more effectively to hold the graft in position. Indeed, micropore tape has a most useful role in minor hand injuries, particularly in children where it can sometimes obviate the need for an anaesthetic of any kind.

The flap has its main use where there has been loss of skin and pulp but where bone and nail are undamaged. The more bone has been lost the less good will be the result. In certain guillotine injuries advancement of the remaining pulp skin distally in the form of a V-shaped flap can be used to close the defect. The method and its indications are discussed on page 266.

A finger tip injury which occurs sufficiently often to constitute a distinct injury pattern is the partially avulsed finger tip which is left attached by a pedicle of pulp. When the injury is of the crushing type the nail is usually avulsed from its base with the flap; the ungual process of the phalanx may be intact but denuded, or fractured with the distal fragment as part of the avulsed segment. With a cutting type of injury the nail may be cut transversely, the distal half remaining attached to the avulsed flap.

It is astonishing how small the pedicle need be to ensure survival of the avulsed flap and a decision as to viability should only be made when the flap has been replaced in its correct position to eliminate the adverse effect of torsion and angulation of the pedicle on the blood supply of the flap. If it is not viable treatment is as for a guillotine amputation. With a viable flap the finger tip should be reconstituted after minimal excision of wound edges and damaged pulp fat. The nail should be retained and replaced in its bed to provide splintage and to ensure a smooth nail bed after healing. In this way the likelihood of distortion when the fresh nail grows in is reduced. When the nail has been transected care should be taken to get the edges accurately apposed for the same reason.

Many finger tip injuries, which ideally should be treated in one of the ways indicated, are of course allowed to heal spontaneously and it is remarkable how well most of them do. This applies most of all to children where the defect in any case is a small one and fear of a tender scar is no problem. This fact indeed should make the surgeon chary about carrying out elaborate procedures at all in children with finger tip injuries. It is astonishing too how, with growth, the scar of a finger tip injury left untreated in the young child shrinks in size and similar shrinkage of a split-skin graft takes place. With this fact in mind there is much to be said for using a thin split skin graft in the hope of maximal shrinkage.

THE ASSOCIATED FRACTURE

A fracture as part of a finger injury adds weight to the argument in favour of amputation, particularly if there is severe comminution. Before such a finger is retained skin cover must be demonstrably available and if it is not available the finger should be amputated unless damage to the remainder of the hand makes retention imperative. As already emphasised the thumb is an exception to this general rule.

If such a finger is retained, the fracture and the soft tissue damage which inevitably accompanies it worsens the prognosis as regards function and adds to the problems of treatment. If the periosteum on either flexor or extensor surface has been extensively damaged by displaced bony fragments there is corresponding damage to the surface over which the tendons move and adhesions rapidly develop between the two surfaces.

Internal fixation by small plate or intramedullary bone peg has been recommended but good results can be achieved by relatively simple methods without recourse to such fixation. The criterion of success is function rather than anatomical perfection of bony contour. With the skin closed the fracture should be reduced and the finger immobilised in the position of function. Plaster of Paris is not always necessary; bulk of dressing often provides entirely adequate splinting.

The problem of subsequent care is to reconcile the needs of the fracture and those of the soft tissues. Immobilisation for the periods usually recommended for closed fractures means a stiff finger and at the end of that period the mature tendon adhesions added to the scarring of other soft tissues makes subsequent mobilisation virtually impossible. A compromise is necessary and it is our experience that by the end of a week to ten days the fracture is sufficiently 'sticky' to permit gentle active exercises within the painless range of movement. Movements are progressively increased at the end of the second week and by the end of the third week a full regime of exercises can be instituted.

When dressings are still required for the skin component of the injury these should be as light as possible to allow the maximum of unhindered movement. In this situation 'Tubegauz' is most useful in providing good cover with a minimum of restraint from sheer bulk of dressing.

ELECTIVE SURGERY

Plastic surgical principles apply also in elective surgery of the hand, both in the surgery of approach to deeper structures and in reconstruction following injury, congenital anomaly, etc.

The placing of scars is important in the surgery of approach, but it has a much wider application in relation to grafts and flaps and will be discussed in relation to all three. In the late reconstruction of the injured hand the problems of skin cover are similar to those of the acute phase and are usually concerned either with skin replacement following excision of contractures and scar or provision of skin cover to permit reconstruction of deep structures, most often tendons. The use of free skin grafts and flaps will be considered both for the primary treatment and the late reconstruction.

The Z-plasty may be required as a secondary procedure where the principles of scar placement have not been followed at the time of primary repair because of precarious blood supply, etc., but it is required all too often to correct the contracted scars resulting from wanton disregard of these principles.

TECHNIQUES OF REPAIR

Suturing techniques

The skin of the palm has strikingly different characteristics from most other sites and these affect its reaction to suture materials. There is a marked tendency when many of the standard materials are used for epithelium to grow along the track of the suture so that when the suture is removed, even relatively soon after insertion, a cone-shaped keratin plug remains like a comedo in the path of the suture. Such a keratin plug can give rise to discomfort amounting to pain on pressure locally, with slight reddening around it, and the condition is slow to subside. Different materials vary in their proneness to this complication, nylon being among the less prone.

The hand, too, is one of the sites where catgut used as a skin suture has a place. Epithelial downgrowth and plug formation do not appear to occur with catgut and, used in children to suture grafts in position and for tie-over bolus dressings, the fact that it dissolves spontaneously saves much heart-burning for the surgeon and his small patients in the subsequent management of their grafts and wounds.

Placing scars in the hand
The major palmar and digital creases indicate lines of flexion in various hand positions and incisions directly across them at right angles should be avoided (Fig. 8.4) as contraction of the scar is liable to cause a flexion contracture.

This principle applies also to grafts and flaps at least to the extent that the margin of the graft or flap should not run in an unbroken line at right angles across a crease. With a graft such a marginal scar is especially liable to contract, as in most cases failure of the graft at its margin for even a millimetre or two produces a scar which gives rise to a contracture. If a straight marginal line is necessary for any reason it will probably require subsequent revision with a Z-plasty inset to break the line.

In the finger the lack of skin wrinkling along the lateral line shows it to be neutral as regards skin tension (Fig. 8.5) and grafts and flaps are best carried well round on to the side of the finger to bring the marginal scar into this neutral line where a minor contracture is of no consequence. When a contracted scar is being excised this may mean that normal skin has to be removed lest contraction of the marginal scar recreate the deformity the procedure was designed to relieve.

Conversely, when the side of the finger is grafted in syndactyly the marginal scar, originally anterolateral, tends with flexion of the finger over a period to move anteriorly further away from the neutral line and forms a contracture requiring a Z-plasty. It is well recognised that incisions along the middle of the palmar aspect of a finger are contra-indicated in general, but given such a scar, a Z-plasty can alleviate at least the contractural result.

Although these rules of scar placement as they relate to the skin creases and the neutral line were accepted *in toto* until recently, it is

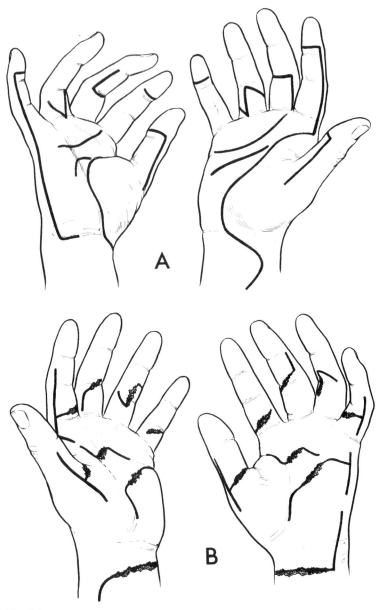

Fig. 8.4

A Commonly used incisions in the hand. These may be combined or modified if necessary with the proviso that the blood supply of any flap raised must be adequate for its survival (after Furlong).

B Suitable incisions extending existing wounds to permit exploration and repair if necessary of nerves and tendons (after Rank and Wakefield).

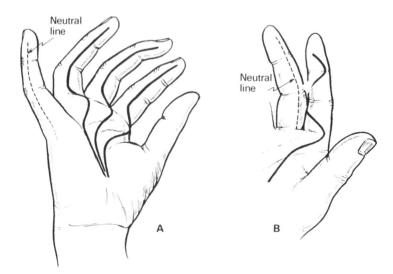

Fig. 8.5 Incisions, as described (A) by Littler and (B) by Bruner, which, although not quite following the restrictive *dicta* illustrated in Figure 8.4, are entirely acceptable. The lateral line having no wrinkling of the skin is neutral for skin tension.

now recognised they are unnecessarily restrictive. Incision lines which appear to transgress the *dicta* outlined above have been found in practice to be perfectly acceptable and indeed are widely used. They either cross the creases at an acute angle or at the neutral line but between the creases they can be allowed to run in virtually any direction. Frequently used examples are shown in Figure 8.5 and the scars following proper use of the multiple Z-plasty also provide examples of these less restrictive practices.

Use of the Z-plasty

Contractures. The Z-plasty has its main value in the well-defined, fairly narrow, linear contracture. The diffuse broad contracture requires the importation of skin by flap or graft.

Where the contracture crosses more than one skin crease a multiple Z-plasty is generally required with a Z to correspond to each crease. As was explained in chapter 2 the lengthening which occurs with each Z is accompanied by transverse shortening and in the hand the amount of transverse slack available is extremely limited. A good working rule is that a Z-plasty of a size which would fit into the adjoining phalangeal segments can be used. This is certainly the largest that should be used and often a smaller one is preferable. The standard 60° Z-plasty is used routinely with the modified flap shape as shown in Figure 2.10 to broaden the tip of each flap. Each Z-plasty can be designed separately if desired; alternatively, and indeed more often, they are planned as a continuous multiple Z-plasty. It is possible to make the multiple Z's skew or symmetrical but unless the presence of previous scarring makes the skew design essential the symmetrical design is much to be preferred.

The elective lines for scars in the hand have already been discussed and it is possible to design the Z-plasties so that, completed, the suture lines lie entirely along elective lines. The key line is the transverse limb of the completed Z-plasty and it must be made to lie in a skin crease.

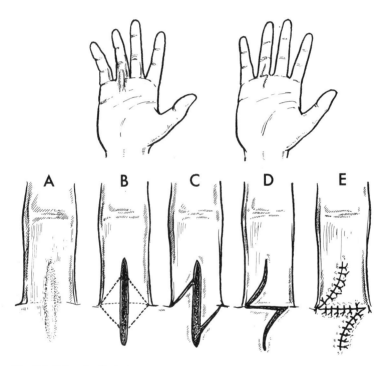

Fig. 8.6 Siting the Z-plasty.

A shows the scar and B the triangles constructed on each side with the intended transverse limb along the metacarpophalangeal joint skin crease. In C the Z-plasty cuts have been selected and made and D shows the flaps transposed. E shows the transposed flaps sutured in position with the transverse limb lying along the skin crease as planned.

To do this the Z-plasty must be planned formally (Fig. 8.6) and drawn out on the skin. The line of the skin crease is marked on the skin with Bonney's Blue as a first step. If, in planning the actual Z-plasty incisions, each is made to end on this line, transposition of the flaps will automatically leave the transverse limb lying along the skin crease as planned.

With the skin crease marked out on the skin, an equilateral triangle can be drawn on each side of the scar into which the Z-plasty is being inserted so that the apex of each triangle is on the skin crease

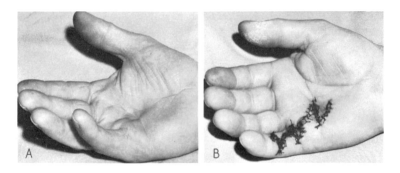

Fig. 8.7 A continuous multiple Z-plasty used in Dupuytren's contracture confined to the little finger ray.
The stages of the procedure are shown diagrammatically in Figure 8.8.

already marked. Of the two possible pairs of Z-plasty flaps outlined in this way the appropriate one can be chosen in the knowledge that as each incision ends on the skin crease completion of the Z-plasty will leave the transverse limb along the skin crease.

When a multiple Z-plasty is used in the hand there is nearly always a redundancy of skin in running from one Z to the next. The temptation to trim this to greater neatness should be resisted. Skin is never available to excess in the palm and, in any case, if the Z's have been planned as recommended the excess will have developed between the skin creases, in the middle of a phalangeal segment. There is a natural bulk in this part of the normal finger and the redundancy settles with time to a normal and natural looking bulkiness.

With the current conservative trend in Dupuytren's contracture where only fascia which is actually contracted is excised, the virtues of the Z-plasty have become increasingly obvious (Fig. 8.7). So often the contracture mainly involves a single ray, palm and finger, presenting clinically as a long linear contracture. The continuous multiple Z-plasty (Fig. 8.8) then has the dual effect of providing ample access to the fascia itself and also of positively relieving any skin contracture or tendency to subsequent scar contraction.

Web deepening. In minor degrees of syndactyly or postburn webbing the Z-plasty can be applied to the problem of deepening the web (Fig. 8.9). If the web is looked on as a line of contracture a Z-plasty can be carried out with a dorsal and a palmar flap. Lengthening the web in this way has the effect of deepening it.

Incidentally such a Z gives excellent exposure of the deep structures of the web; it allows, for example, the superficial transverse ligament of the palmar aponeurosis to be excised easily when it is severely involved in Dupuytren's contracture.

USE OF FREE SKIN GRAFTS

In a difficult situation where take of a graft is likely to be hazardous, as with a granulating surface or in primary trauma, the overriding need is for successful take and the split-skin graft is therefore the graft of choice regardless of site. Even in the palm of hand and finger where secondary contracture is inevitable it must still be used, to be replaced if necessary by a whole skin graft at a later date when conditions for take are better.

It is in the uncrushed injury that grafts take most easily; in the crush injury they take much less well. Crushing probably produces devitalisation of the tissues severe enough to effect adversely the vacularisation of a graft yet insufficient to jeopardise the viability of the finger as a whole. Recognition of this fact suggests the desirability, where possible, of more radical debridement of the recipient site in preparation for the graft in crushing injuries.

In elective surgery and the secondary repair of hand injuries graft usage differs in dorsum and palm. The split-skin graft, preferably thick, can be used on the dorsum; on the palm between the fingers, and in the webs, where secondary contracture would so often destroy the whole point of the procedure, a whole skin graft is generally preferable.

There is a tendency for a line of contraction to develop at the margin of a graft, whether whole skin or split-skin, by a process akin to that which causes scar contraction. The degree of contraction and the resulting contracture may be minimal or severe depending on how rapidly marginal healing has taken place. While it is not always possible to avoid such contraction its more severe effects can at least be mitigated by placing the margin of the graft along one of the elective incision lines already described (p. 247). The bringing of the graft margin to such a line may of course mean carrying the graft

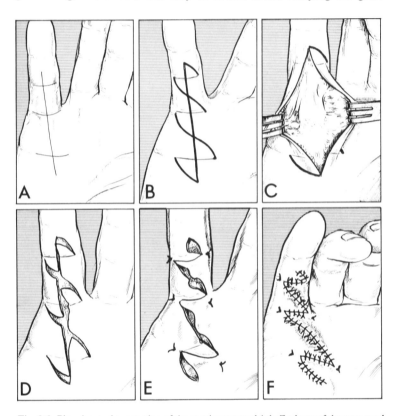

Fig. 8.8 Planning and excecution of the continuous multiple Z-plasty of the type used in the Dupuytren's contracture shown in Figure 8.7. The line of the long incision indicating the extent of the contracted fascia and the intended lines of the transverse limbs of the Z-plasty is shown (A). B shows the Z-plasty drawn to place the transverse limbs in the creases as planned (see Fig. 8.6). The good exposure obtained by the longitudinal incision is seen C. D shows the Z-plasty flaps incised, transposed for suture, E, and sutured, F.

beyond the obvious defect, if need be excising normal skin to do so. If this is felt to be undesirable, the alternative may be to break the line of any contracture which subsequently develops with a Z-plasty.

The method of applying and suturing the graft is similar to that described for general use. When applying the tie-over flavine wool

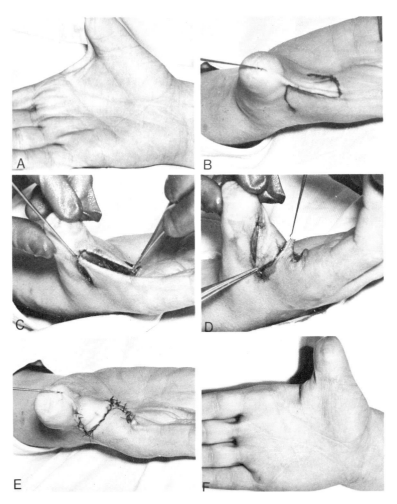

Fig. 8.9 The use of a Z-plasty in deepening the web between the thumb and index finger to increase the grasp of a thumb short as a result of trauma.

and the subsequent pressure dressing care should be taken to avoid undue pressure on the graft. It is the graft on dorsum of fingers and hand which is specially liable to be adversely affected by too much pressure and the prominences caused by the heads of the metacarpals and proximal phalanges are the most vulnerable areas. Over these areas too graft failure is most serious for exposure of tendon and joint capsule is the inevitable result. The prominences are increased by marked flexion of the fingers and so the hand should be immobilised, if anything, on the extended side of the position of function.

The application of the dressing will be discussed under the heading of postoperative care.

USE OF FLAPS

Different sources of skin vary in the extent to which they reproduce the characteristics of the skin of the defect in texture and appearance, etc., but this aspect is only one of the factors to be considered in an individual case and not always the most important. The appropriate type of flap, its source, etc., tends to be governed more by the size of the defect and its site.

The flaps available are **local** and **distant**. Local flaps of the transposed or rotation type have an extremely limited role because the defect which can be covered by the size of flap which the hand is capable of providing is of necessity such a very small one. Cross-finger and thenar flaps, though local in a sense, have the characteristics of the distant flaps and should really be classed with them. In any case they will be discussed later.

Until recently distant flaps were restricted to direct or tubed pedicle flaps, and each had its advantages and limitations. The direct flap was capable of being used primarily, that is without preliminary delay, and was consequently suitable for use in acute trauma; the tube pedicle required preliminary preparation before it could be applied to a hand and this ruled it out for use in acute trauma. The tube pedicle had the advantage of requiring comparatively little preliminary planning because of the latitude which its long pedicle permitted; the very short pedicle of the direct flap reduced the margin for error very greatly and it had to be planned with great care. The advent of the axial pattern flaps has made both largely superfluous (Figs. 4.35 and 4.37). The highly favourable length–breadth ratio possible with all three, deltopectoral, groin and hypogastric, reduces the need for careful positional planning and fixation. At the same time the lack of need for prior preparation means that they are available for use in acute trauma.

Which of the three flaps should be used in a particular clinical situation will depend on various factors. In favour of the deltopectoral flap is the thinness of the flap, the lack of dependence of the hand and the comfort of the position it has to take up, though against this, in the short, broad chested patient particularly, the position may call for an undesirable degree of elbow flexion. Used in acute trauma, the flexion of the elbow required to maintain position may accentuate any tendency to traumatic oedema. At the same time, the site of the secondary defect may be undesirable especially in the female (Fig. 8.10).

The groin and the hypogastric flaps have features in common and are equally suitable in many instances. It may be felt that the degree of dependency of the hand inseparable from their use will give rise to oedema but this has not proved so in practice. It has been found that, *provided a full regimen of regular exercises is instituted*, oedema

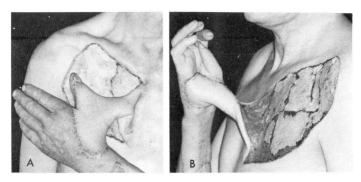

Fig. 8.10 Examples of the deltopectoral flap, used to resurface (A) the dorsal and (B) the palmar surface of the hand. The length of the pedicle and the consequent freedom of movement possible is seen.

does not occur. The position of the hand with either flap is a comfortable one, but the hypogastric flap transfers skin which is often hairy while the groin flap uses skin usually free of hair even in the most hirsute. Both sites can be undesirably fat, the hypogastrium more so than the flank, and this might influence the surgeon in his choice. The secondary defect of the groin flap is the least conspicuous of the three and can almost always be closed by direct suture.

In preparing the recipient site for a flap of any kind the margin should always be excised to healthy tissue and this applies with special force to a granulating area, for only with radical excision can the flap be soundly sutured to good surgical material. As has been pointed out in relation both to scars and free skin grafts in the hand, and for the same reasons, the margin between a flap and the hand is best placed along one of the elective lines for scars. To achieve this it may be necessary to bring the flap beyond the obvious defect.

It is usually possible to tube the pedicle of an axial pattern flap but it is seldom possible to raise a reception flap in the hand when a direct flap is used and the split-skin graft covering the donor site of the flap must be extended to line the bridge segment.

When a flap is being transferred as a preliminary to a reconstructive procedure, e.g. of tendon, it is usually advisable to have the transfer complete and the area quite healed before the deep structure is treated so that the possibility of sepsis can be eliminated.

Defects proximal to the webs

If a defect of the dorsum is small a rotation or transposed flap is occasionally a possible method of repair (Fig. 8.11). The amount of 'slack' available on the dorsum is deceptively small and free skin grafting of the secondary defect is almost universally needed. In practice, cases suitable for a local flap seldom occur and in particular the temptation to use a local flap in the older age group should be strongly resisted. Ageing, atrophic skin does badly as a flap and necrosis is apt to occur. Rotation flaps of the palm cannot be recommended from any point of view because of the characteristics of the skin itself and its intimate attachment to the palmar aponeurosis.

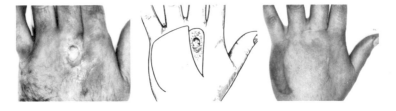

Fig. 8.11 Defect of the dorsum of the hand resulting from an electrical burn with loss of extensor tendon. The transposed flap used to provide cover permitted subsequent tendon repair by extensor indicis transfer.

In deciding the appropriate source for a flap much depends on the size of the defect. For the defect of intermediate size near the radial or ulnar side a direct flap from the opposite forearm is a possibility, and the upper arm is also a source. This latter source had been used effectively in the adduction contracture of the first web to provide a flap for the web itself. The hand fits particularly well around the upper arm and the position is a comfortable one.

The problem which must be faced and accepted by the patient with a cross-arm flap is his inability to look after his toilet requirements and this is a very real factor in limiting its value.

For the larger defect one of the axial pattern flaps is the method to use (Fig. 8.12).

Defects distal to the webs
The defect may be of one finger only or of several fingers and according to circumstances a **distant** flap from trunk, or a **local** flap from the same or an adjoining finger or thenar eminence may be used for cover.

Distant flaps
When a single finger is involved the decision of whether or not a trunk flap can be used depends largely on the site of the defect for the other fingers may make it impossible to bring the defect and potential flap together readily. It is more for pulp replacement that a trunk flap is used though even here skin more near in character to normal pulp skin is preferable where a suitable flap can be constructed.

Defects of several fingers may be dealt with simultaneously by suturing the adjacent margin of each defect so that one large defect is made which can then be covered with a single flap (Fig. 8.13). When the fingers come subsequently to be separated it will be found that the amount of skin needed for each finger is greater than one might have expected. The thickness of the flap makes this unavoidable even allowing for as much thinning as possible and the flap should be of correspondingly generous dimensions. The subsequent separation of the fingers and thinning of the flaps can be a prolonged and tiresome process, of necessity carried out in stages, and an alternative, if somewhat drastic, approach is to excise the flap completely and replace it with a free skin graft. While the fact that the original defect was unsuitable for free skin grafting may have provided the reason for using the flap in the first place, careful removal of the flap subsequently should leave a defect which can be grafted successfully.

At what point in time the flap should be replaced with the graft is a matter of judgment in the individual case. The earliest is probably 10 days after the flap has been applied, but replacement can be deferred until the 21st day, the usual time for dividing a flap. The flap then, instead of having its pedicle divided, can be raised and returned to its donor site. Alternatively, division and insetting can

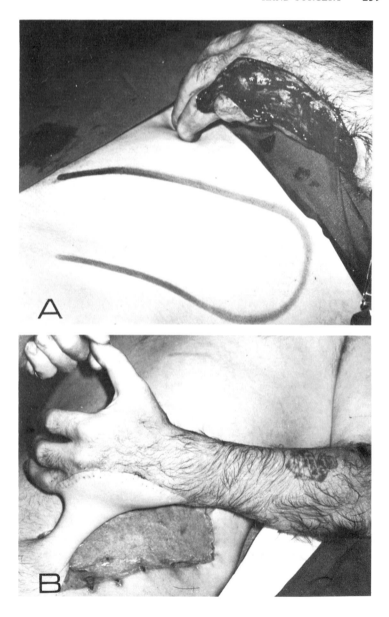

Fig. 8.12 The groin flap used to resurface a defect of the ulnar side of the hand.

A   The defect and the flap drawn out.

B   The flap raised and transferred, its bridge segment tubed.

In this instance the secondary defect was split-skin grafted, but greater experience has shown that most defects can be closed by direct suture.

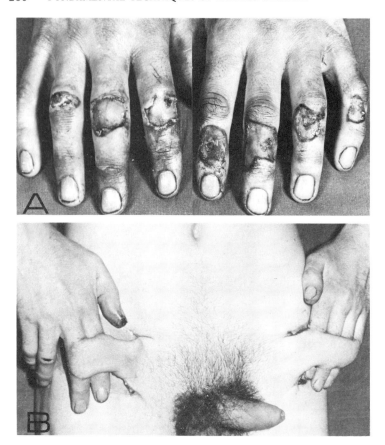

Fig. 8.13 The conversion of an injury of several fingers into a single defect prior to flap cover and the use of the groin flap to provide flap cover. The injury (A) of the dorsum of several fingers of each hand, total skin loss burns with underlying extensor expansion damage, converted into single defects and covered with bilateral groin flaps. The subsequent management of this patient is shown in Fig. 8.14.

be completed and excision of the flap postponed until any lingering stiffness of the fingers has gone (Fig. 8.14).

For the defect of intermediate size the cross-arm flap from the other forearm is a possible method of covering either the dorsal or palmar surface of a finger. The position is easy to maintain and the flap can be of the direct type if the length–breadth ratio permits. When the ratio makes such a flap risky the bipedicled strap flap may be used instead. The flexor aspect of the forearm is the obvious donor site but as long as the flap does not encroach on the

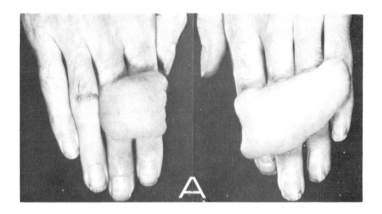

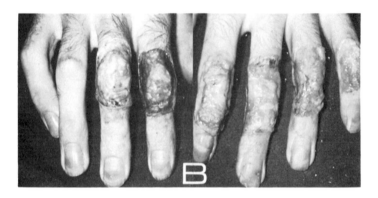

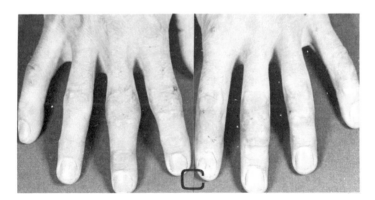

Fig. 8.14 The management of the flap applied to several fingers, as shown in Fig. 8.13. (A) shows the groin flaps divided to allow the earliest possible full mobilisation of the hand, elbow and shoulder, leaving the temporary syndactyly, (B) shows the surface left following excision of the flap from each hand, ready for grafting and (C) shows the end result following split-skin grafting.

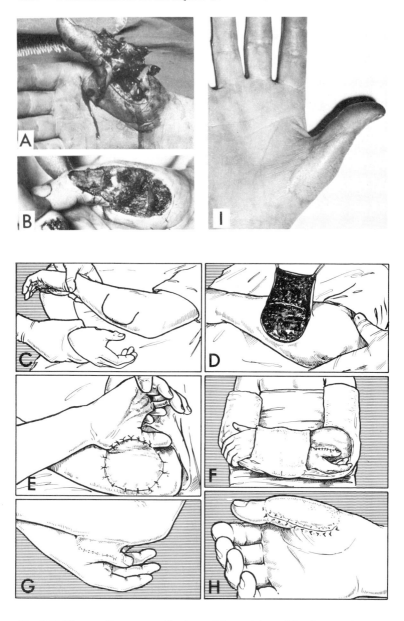

Fig. 8.15 The use of a cross-arm flap in repairing an injury of the thenar eminence. The injury (A), involving the metacarpophalangeal joint, prepared (B) to receive the flap. The flap outlined (C), and raised (D). The split-skin graft applied to the secondary defect showing the extension of the graft to line the pedicle segment of the flap (E) and the plaster of Paris fixation of the arms (F). The flap immediately before division (G), and divided and inset (H). The final result (I).

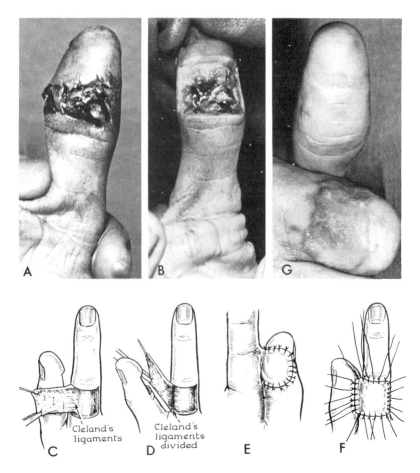

Fig. 8.16 A cross-finger flap used to resurface the pulp of thumb. The injury (A), prepared to receive the flap (B). The flap raised before (C), and after (D), incising Cleland's ligaments, and sutured in position (E) with split-skin graft applied to the secondary defect (F). The final result (G).

subcutaneous border of the ulna any site which permits a comfortable position during transfer may be used (Fig. 8.15). While the cross-arm flap is undoubtedly a possible method the nursing problems associated with it make it, as already stressed, a method to have in reserve rather than one to be used routinely.

Local flaps
These can be taken from an adjoining finger or the thenar eminence as cross-finger and thenar flaps. Certain finger tip injuries can also

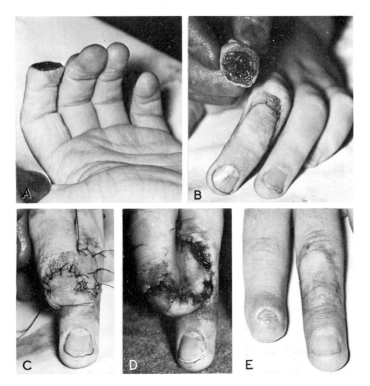

Fig. 8.17 The distally based cross-finger flap used to cover a guillotined index finger-tip. The injury (A) and the flap (B), sutured in positon with a split-skin graft applied to the secondary defect (C). The dressing 14 days later (D), and the end result (E).

This is a common injury and when the preservation of length of the finger is considered desirable the flap is a most useful one. The distal basing of the flap does not jeopardise its viability.

be managed by advancing the pulp skin distally using the V–Y principle.

Cross-finger flap (Fig. 8.16 and 8.17). This type of flap can provide cover for a defect of the palmar aspect of a finger, particularly in the middle and proximal phalangeal segments, since it can only be taken from the dorsum and side of the donor finger. It is most useful for defects of between one and two phalangeal segments. Smaller defects increase the length–breadth ratio while the technical difficulties increase if the area to be covered is much longer than this. The flap finds one of its most effective uses in covering the thumb.Whether pulp or tip is being covered the thumb can readily be positioned so that the flap from index finger is not under tension and its pedicle is not subject to undue torsion.

The flap must be raised with care to avoid baring the digital nerve and artery or extensor expansion and the secondary defect on the donor finger is covered with a thick split-skin graft.

The reach of a cross-finger flap can be increased if a point is made of dividing Cleland's skin ligaments. These ligaments as they appear in this surgical procedure form a fibrous septum just dorsal to the neurovascular bundle and bind the skin of the neutral line to the side of each phalanx. Their division frees the skin of the neutral line and adds greatly to the mobility and reach of the flap itself.

A modification of the cross-finger flap as described can be used to resurface the tip of a finger when the relative lengths of donor and recipient fingers are suitable and the mobility of the recipient finger adequate (Fig. 8.17). It is important to avoid encroaching on the nail bed of the donor finger when the flap is constructed. The index finger is the one which most often sustains an injury requiring this particular flap.

Thenar flap. It is well recognised that flexion of any of the four fingers brings its pulp to almost the same point of the thenar eminence and this fact can be used in resurfacing pulp or finger tip defects by a flap raised on the thenar eminence (Fig. 8.18). The flap has its main use in the hand with relatively thin palmar skin; the calloused hand of the manual worker is quite unsuited for the procedure. If the patient is unable to bring the finger requiring cover to lie against the thenar eminence easily and with a complete absence of discomfort the flap should never be contemplated. This excludes it as a rule from being considered for the index and little fingers.

The dimensions and site of the defect determine how the flap should be based. For a defect of the greater part of the pulp a side-based flap offers the best length-breadth ratio. The secondary defect is covered with a thick split-skin graft.

Planning with jaconet, so effective elsewhere, does not work well with the thenar flap. The bloodstained imprint of the flexed finger is more useful in giving the appropriate site and shape of the flap to be raised.

This flap has its enthusiastic advocates though these are now much fewer in number and the flap is certainly not without unsatisfactory aspects. A tender scar in the thenar area is a serious disability and occasionally occurs, and the finger immobilised in flexion for the period necessary is sometimes difficult to mobilise. In addition it is difficult to avoid maceration of skin in the operative site from the close proximity of flap and palm for the area sweats

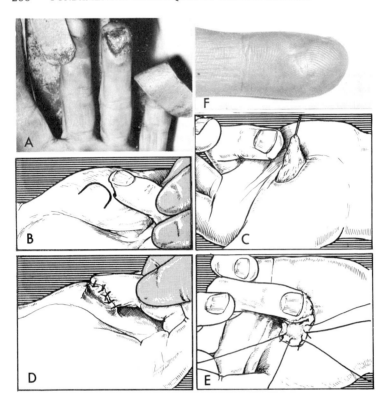

Fig. 8.18 The use of a thenar flap to repair a defect (A) of pulp of finger. The flap is outlined with Bonney's Blue (B) on the thenar eminence, elevated (C) and sutured to the defect (D). A split-skin graft is sutured to the secondary defect (E), the sutures being left long for the tie-over dressing. The final result after division of the pedicle and insetting of the flap is shown (F).

virtually continuously at ordinary temperatures. Shortly after it was first described it was widely used, probably in many instances when its use was ill-advised, and its popularity has undoubtedly waned. Recently a modified version has been described in which the flap is raised from the region of the metacarpophalangeal skin crease of the thumb, an area felt less likely to give trouble from a tender scar than the thenar eminence. This modification, though an improvement, does not really eliminate the other unsatisfactory aspects of the method. It remains a flap to use sparingly and only when the indications are clear.

V—Y flap (Fig. 8.19). Following a guillotine amputation it may be possible to cover the finger tip defect by advancing distally a

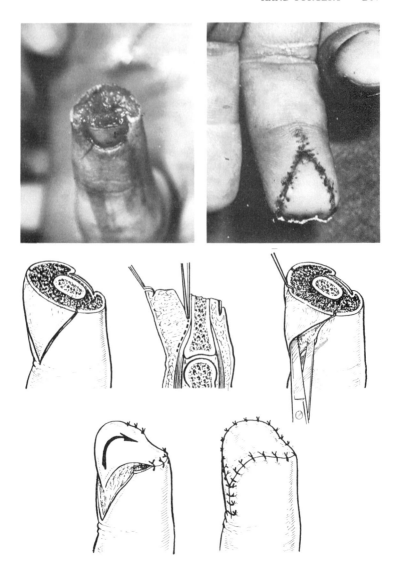

Fig. 8.19 The V-Y flap as applied to the guillotine amputation of finger tip, showing the various stages of the method.

V-shaped flap of the pulp skin, approximating the skin on either side to close the residual pulp defect. The effect is to convert the initial V of the flap into a Y-shaped suture line.

The V is designed on the pulp skin so that its apex reaches almost to the distal interphalangeal crease and the width of its base distally should equal that of the nail. The incision along the limbs of the V goes through skin alone. Thereafter, sharp-pointed scissors thrust carefully into the pulp fat and gently opened mobilise the flap without destroying its nerve and vascular attachment to the proximal finger. Freeing of the flap deeply is carried out by dividing its fibrous attachment to the distal phalanx and the distal fibrous flexor sheath close to these structures. Mobilised, the flap is advanced distally and sutured to the margins of the pulp defect with fine sutures. Suturing around each side of the flap proceeds until the lines meet at the apex of the V and continues proximally, converting the suture line into a Y.

Two conditions must be met before the method is indicated. No element of devitalising crushing must exist and enough pulp must remain to provide a flap of adequate size. The appropriate injury for the method is the oblique slicing injury whose obliquity leaves more pulp than nail.

Sensory factors in the use of flaps

A factor in assessing the value of these various flaps and one which has not received the emphasis it deserves is the sensation which they eventually develop. Different areas of the hand differ in the sensory demands which the patient places on them. The important areas clearly are the pulp segments and the different fingers themselves vary in comparative importance. Thumb and index finger in their normally apposing surfaces, the 'pinch sites', are of prime significance and thereafter importance diminishes from radial to ulnar side of the hand subject to the proviso that the ulnar side of the little finger is comparatively important and the radial side of the other fingers is more important than the ulnar, since this is the side most likely to be used in prehensile movements.

But while these relative importances are true in the normal hand they may have to be appraised afresh in the mutilated hand. The important fact is that they should be assessed, and the assessment reflected in the selection of the donor and recipient sites for any island flap, both from the viewpoint of the finger chosen and the precise site on it.

The return of sensation in flaps is extremely variable and depends, among other things, on the quota of nerve fibres in the bed of the flap and the degree of scarring, both deep and marginal. The functional adequacy of the sensation which does return depends of course on the site and the demands put on it. In the most demanding areas, the pinch sites, the quality of sensation which can be expected to return even at best is not even remotely adequate. It is for this reason among others that the neurovascular island flap has proved such a valuable adjunct to the standard flaps. In areas where tactile discrimination is less important and protective sensation is enough the amount which returns is sufficient. It is wise nevertheless to warn the patient to be careful and avoid burning the flap while it is anaesthetic.

POSTOPERATIVE CARE

Following a surgical procedure in the hand a period of immobilisation is generally desirable and this is provided by the dressing on occasion reinforced by plaster of Paris. At the same time measures should be taken to prevent oedema developing in the hand.

Dressing of the hand

If a graft has been applied it is usually wise, regardless of the site of the graft, to immobilise the entire hand in the position of function. Following the tie-over dressing careful padding of the whole hand, in the webs and between the fingers, must be carried out before applying the circumferential crepe bandages. The aim in padding is to convert the hand into a cylinder so that pressure is evenly distributed. Failure to pad the palm and dorsum adequately causes undue pressure on the radial and ulnar sides and sores may result. Only the finger tips are left visible to indicate the vascular state of the hand.

When no graft has been used absolute immobilisation may be less necessary and the regime can be suitably relaxed.

The 'position of function' in fact needs to be defined in a little more detail in relation to hand surgery. It is now generally recognised that the hand immobilised for any length of time regains a full range of joint movement faster and more readily if it has been immobilised with the metacarpo-phalangeal joints flexed and the interphalangeal joints extended—a position one might call the 'position of immobilisation'. When a hand is to be fixed for three weeks it should thus be in the position of immobilisation. Fortunately, when a graft has been applied, fixation is never for as long as three weeks and the position can safely be modified to suit the needs of the graft. In particular the metacarpophalangeal joint can be extended and somewhat to avoid the undue prominence of the metacarpal head and consequent vulnerability from too much local pressure.

The positioning of the hand to get a flap to lie properly may equally be unsuitable from a joint point of view and this has to be accepted as a hazard. Nevertheless, awareness of the fact that the ideal position has been departed from will remind the surgeon to keep the less than ideal position for the shortest possible time and redouble his encouragement to subsequent mobilisation of the joints.

Prevention of oedema

Oedema fluid provides the raw material of stiff fingers and is prevented by elevation. Various methods are used (Fig. 8.20). A well padded plaster of Paris cast encircling the arm as far proximally as the upper humerus, so that weight is taken on the upper arm and not on the wrist and hand, may be used but its weight tends to be resented by the patient.

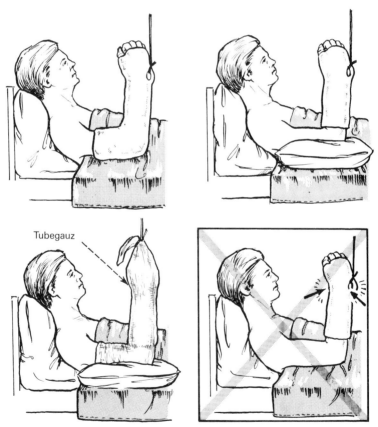

Tubegauz

Fig. 8.20 Various methods of postoperatively elevating the hand. Note how the incorrect method produces constriction distal to the wrist.

Alternatively the plaster may be confined to below the elbow and the elbow supported on a pillow, suspension merely keeping it vertical. Suspension with 'Tubegauz' works well and it can be continued up the arm to the axilla so that any traction is spread as widely as possible.

Whatever the method the plaster must not be allowed to hang free and constrict the wrist. In more minor procedures elevation on a pillow or in a sling without plaster of Paris is adequate. The sling should be such that the hand is as high as is consistent with comfort.

When a distant flap has been applied to the hand, elevation is naturally not possible. Its role as a prophylactic against oedema must then be replaced by a vigorous regimen of active exercises, every joint not of necessity immobilised being regularly put through a full range. If such a regimen is applied dependency will not be found to create problems.

Subsequent dressings

Unless there is a good reason most dressings in hand injuries should be left untouched for a week and many can safely be left for longer. The less the injury and dressings are interfering with hand function the less the need for early dressing and, if there are no clinical signs to suggest infection, the first dressing can often be left until the tenth to twelfth day. This applies even to the injury involving a graft. When the function of the hand is significantly limited by the dressings, particularly in older patients, the first dressing should generally be done on the seventh day and the bulk of dressings thereafter should be reduced to a minimum so that movement of the fingers can be instituted as rapidly and intensively as possible.

A similar approach applies to the dressing following elective procedures.

9

Surgery of the eyelids

Skin cover of the eyelids is usually required as a result of loss from trauma or surgical excision for malignancy.

EYELID INJURIES

The extremely rich blood supply of the eyelids permits survival of flaps with the most tenuous of attachments. It follows that the approach to the treatment of trauma in this region must be ultra-conservative; wound excision should be minimal and the surgeon's chief aim should be to replace tissues in their proper anatomical site (Fig. 9.1). The severely damaged eyelid may present a veritable jigsaw puzzle, but reassembling the various parts correctly is not labour wasted; even if secondary operations are required to correct skin or deep contractures they will be easy and successful in direct proportion to the care taken and the accuracy achieved at the primary operation.

When an eyelid injury is first seen there often appears to be actual loss of tissue but the true loss can be assessed only as the repair proceeds and is almost always less than at first seemed likely. In repairing these injuries there are certain key structures which, correctly placed as a first step, can act as landmarks.

Tear duct system. When the lower lid canaliculus has been severed, it is desirable to reconstitute it where possible. Failure to do so may result in an intractable epiphora and late reconstruction is not possible. A careful search should be made for the cut end leading to the lacrimal sac, but if it cannot be found, passage of a nylon thread or probe through the canaliculus of the intact lid and lacrimal sac will sometimes help in identifying it (Fig. 9.1). In the same way, if the segment in the lid cannot be seen, passage of a nylon or silkworm gut thread through the punctum will show the cut end of the canaliculus where it emerges. Passage of the thread into the other orifice will allow healing in continuity. This procedure is easier to describe than carry out but it is worth attempting where possible.

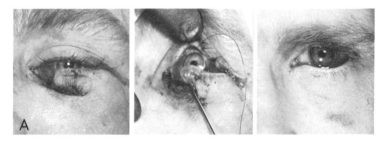

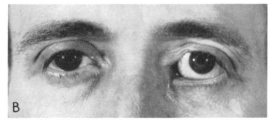

Fig. 9.1

A Repair of an injury without tissue loss avulsing the lower lid from its medial attachment, showing an attempt to restore the continuity of the canaliculus by threading monofilament nylon through the lacrimal punctum and into the lacrimal sac.

The final result shows the excellent appearance which can be achieved by accurate reconstitution of the medial canthus.

B The result of failure to reconstruct the canthus accurately following an injury similar to A.

The repair of an injury similar to A as part of a more extensive facial soft tissue injury is shown in Figure 1.2.

The tendency to stricture even when the canaliculus is reconstituted is marked and despite passage of probes drainage of tears is often poor. Fortunately even with complete failure to reconstitute the canaliculus the epiphora is not invariably severe.

Lid margin. Various methods of stepping incisions or wounds of the lid margin have been described but careful matching is quite adequate if the wound edge is made to evert a little by the suture. In any case it would be quite unjustifiable to traumatise still further tissues already damaged by the injury. The various landmarks of the lid margin—the eyelashes, the grey line, the junction of conjunctiva and skin, all can be used for matching purposes.

Tarsal plates. In each eyelid the tarsal plate is closely adherent to the conjunctiva and in trauma the two behave as a single structure. It is advisable where possible to avoid sutures in the conjunctiva but matching of the tarsal plates can be used to fix the margins of the associated conjunctiva which in any case heals very rapidly.

Conjunctiva. At the completion of any repair it is essential to have a situation which will permit cover of the cornea with lid conjunctiva during sleep and a tarsorrhaphy is sometimes needed to ensure this. Sutures in the conjunctiva cause irritation of the cornea where the two come into contact, they are difficult to remove, and are best avoided. When they cannot be avoided, a continuous 'interweaving' suture (Fig. 9.2) brought out to the skin surface at each end is useful. It draws the conjunctiva together well, there is no interlocking, and it is readily removed. The smooth surface of nylon thread can be turned to advantage in this situation for easy removal.

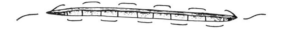

Fig. 9.2 The interweaving suture (after Stallard).

Palpebral ligaments. The tarsal plates which give to the eyelids such rigidity as they possess have their main attachment to the bony orbit via the medial and lateral palpebral ligaments and, if either of these ligaments has been divided traumatically, it must be reconstituted as far as possible by suture. The medial ligament is the more powerful structure and damage to it is correspondingly serious, for the whole medial canthal region drifts forward and laterally giving the appearance of a unilateral hypertelorism. It is stated that this appearance only results if the posterior attachment of the ligament behind the lacrimal sac is divided but, at least as far as trauma is concerned, this is largely an academic point.

Unfortunately it is extremely difficult to reconstitute the ligamentous attachment and though the immediate postoperative position of the lids following wiring, etc., of the ligament to its bony insertion may be good, the system tends to drift back to its pre-operative position.

USE OF GRAFTS

Ideally a graft replacing eyelid skin must fulfil certain requirements which arise from the functional anatomy of the region. Firstly, the lack of rigidity of the normal tarsal plate makes the eyelids prone to cicatricial ectropion or entropion if there is the slightest contracture on the surface of the lid or in the socket. Secondly, eyelid skin is extremely thin and in the upper lid particularly is only loosely attached deeply because of the need for rapid movement of the eyelids. The lower eyelid is less mobile than the upper and the part of the upper lid corresponding to the tarsal plate is in its turn less mobile than that above the upper palpebral furrow.

Skin grafted to an eyelid should be as thin as normal eyelid skin, especially when the most mobile skin is being replaced, and in addition should be free of a tendency to secondary contraction. Unfortunately the best skin, which comes from the upper eyelid, is extremely limited in quantity at best and may not be available at all and so a compromise has generally to be reached (Fig. 9.3). For less mobile areas, the canthi, the lower eyelid and the tarsal segment of the upper eyelid, postauricular whole thickness skin provides the best substitute, gives an excellent colour and texture match, and its extreme vascularity makes take easy.

In the upper part of the upper eyelid, the need for extreme mobility is paramount and a thin split-skin graft from the anterior or medial aspect of the upper arm is usually used. With the knowledge that such a graft will undergo gross secondary contraction, the defect is stretched to its maximum and indeed over-corrected so that the largest possible area of skin can be inserted in expectation of secondary contraction. Despite this, the graft area nearly always does end up a little shorter than normal in the vertical dimension.

Preparation for grafting
Following surgical excision and immediately following trauma, the actual skin defect is already visible, but in the late repair of trauma, the defect usually shows as ectropion and must be demonstrated afresh as a raw surface so that it may be corrected.

If the skin loss has been localised the scarred area is well delineated and can be dealt with, excising the scarring so that the eyelid may lie against the eyeball. When the resulting defect is in the upper part of the upper eyelid and a split-skin graft is felt to be appropriate additional transverse incisions medially and laterally beyond the area of actual scarring are advisable so that the original defect may be overcorrected to allow for the subsequent contraction of the graft. When a postauricular whole skin graft is felt to be adequate such overcorrection is less necessary.

The ectropion which results from a full thickness skin loss burn is more diffuse and to demonstrate the extent of the skin lost a different method is used (Fig. 9.4). With skin hooks on the lid margin to put the skin on the stretch, an incision is made approximately 2 mm on the skin side of the eyelashes and parallel to them. If the contracture has distorted the canthus, and the lateral is the one liable to be pulled off the eyeball, the incision should be prolonged

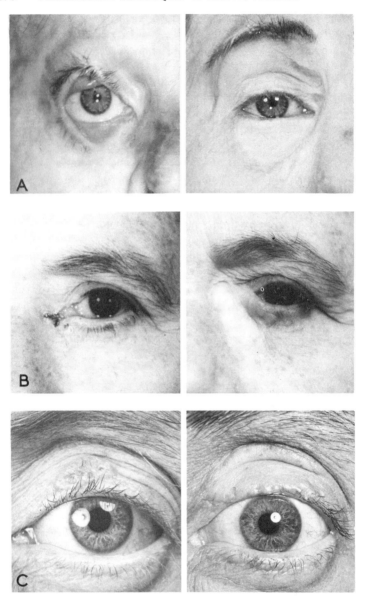

Fig. 9.3 The free skin grafts used in the various eyelid sites.

A   Postburn ectropion of both eyelids. Upper lid skin replaced by split-skin from upper arm and lower eyelid skin replaced by postauricular whole thickness skin.
B   Basal cell carcinoma of medial canthus involving the caruncle and adjoining eyelids replaced after excision by postauricular whole thickness skin.
C   Basal cell carcinoma of skin overlying the upper tarsal plate replaced after excision by postauricular whole thickness skin.

beyond it, so that any skin loss in a transverse as well as a vertical direction may be corrected. An incision confined to the actual lid margin in such circumstances tends to leave slight residual ectropion towards the canthus.

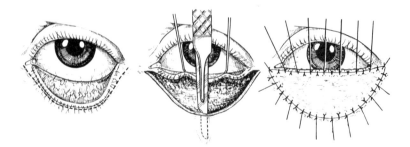

Fig. 9.4 The method of correcting diffuse ectropion of the lower eyelid and the insertion of a postauricular whole skin graft.

Maintaining tension on the hooks, the knife blade is worked away from the lid margin parallel to and just deep to the skin surface separating skin from underlying muscle. As dissection proceeds the ectropion becomes increasingly corrected and the skin defect displayed. The lid should be freed until it lies spontaneously against the eyeball along its entire length and can readily be stretched well over its fellow eyelid. Even after extensive freeing the lid may still tend to lie off the globe and this is generally due to residual areas of scarring in the orbicularis muscle. These patches of scarring are felt rather than seen and must be excised completely with fine scissors. Even what would seem to be a most radical excision of much of the muscle leaves no disability; only if the levator palpebrae superioris is divided will there be ptosis. The undermining of the lid margin for a millimetre or so to give a good suture line completes the preparation for the graft.

The extent of the defect of eyelid made surgically is usually governed by pathological considerations but on occasion additional normal skin has to be excised to give a better line to the junction of graft and surrounding skin. An example of such a situation is the extending of excision a little beyond the canthus, if the junction of graft and surrounding eyelid is approaching it. Also, just as straight vertical scars from the lid margin are best avoided lest contraction of the scar cause ectropion, a vertical junction of graft and eyelid is undesirable. When it is unavoidable, the defect should be fully displayed so that the maximum of skin can be inserted to allow for any subsequent contraction.

The application of the graft
The method of applying a whole skin graft differs only in minor details from elsewhere. It is safer to suture away from the eyeball though this may mean suturing from a less to a more mobile structure and the sutures along the eyelid margin should not be tied too tightly as they cut through readily. In the same way the sutures tied over the flavine wool bolus should not put too much strain on the sutures. Undue pressure is not necessary; these grafts take very readily if haematoma is avoided.

With a split-skin graft the same technique of applying the graft can be used, but the object is to stretch the defect to allow as much skin as possible to be inserted and the flavine wool technique does not lend itself readily to this. The stretching and overcorrection is better achieved using the STENT mould technique (Fig. 9.5). STENT is a dental moulding compound which softens to malleability in hot water and hardens to rigidity in cold and it can be used to take an accurate impression of the stretched defect. The graft is draped over the mould with its raw surface outwards so that it completely covers the surface of the mould which is going to be inserted into the defect. The mould with skin is then laid into the raw area. Sutures through the skin edges of the defect are tied over the mould half burying it so that the maximum contact of raw surface and graft is obtained and in this way the maximum of graft is inserted. There is no question of suturing the graft edge to edge to the defect. Any obvious excess is trimmed off when the tieover sutures are tied, the graft takes to the margin of the defect and at the first dressing, usually seven days later, the skin beyond the edge of the defect, dry and papery by now, is easily trimmed off.

Before the dressing is applied it is always advisable with either technique to 'vaseline' the eyelashes away from the eyeball. To distribute pressure the dressing is built up around the flavine wool or mould and a crepe bandage is applied. Unless it is felt that movement of the eyeball underneath will irritate the cornea, and with a simple graft of skin alone this is seldom true, there is no need to cover the other eye. Some surgeons carry out a temporary tarsorrhaphy simultaneously but this is quite unnecessary.

Postoperative care
Apart from failure of the graft to take, and this fortunately is extremely rare, the only complication to be feared is corneal ulceration and this is usually the result of trichiasis which has not been dealt with immediately. The patient must be specifically asked if he feels anything in his eye and a positive reply is an absolute

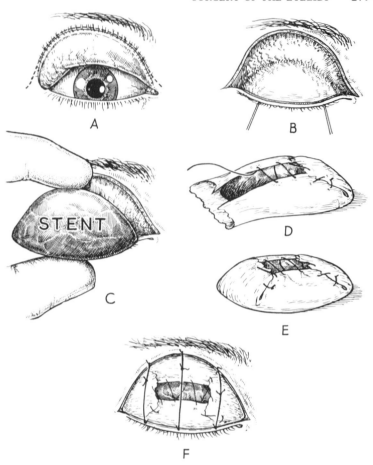

Fig. 9.5 The STENT technique of grafting an eyelid. The ectropion of upper lid (A) is corrected (B) and a STENT mould (C) of the defect is made. The split-skin graft with raw surface outwards is draped round the mould (D and E) and inserted into the defect (F).

indication to take down the dressing and inspect the eye for the offending eyelash. This applies regardless of the consequences to the graft though fortunately take and vascularisation are so rapid that the graft is seldom jeopardised by a careful inspection. Patients occasionally complain of some pain but give a negative reply to the direct question about the feeling of a foreign body. In such cases there is seldom need to take down the dressing; gentle easing of the bandage is usually adequate.

The graft is dressed on the seventh day and a further dressing is often wise for a further week or so, not so much to provide pressure as immobility. The lids are so mobile that even after a 100 per cent take some loss may occur if unlimited lid movements are allowed too soon.

USE OF FLAPS

When a full-thickness defect of eyelid has to be repaired a flap may be necessary for skin cover, but for skin replacement alone it is less often used. Following excision of a malignant lesion, it is not easy to justify its use if skin alone is involved, though on grounds other than pathological it will give an entirely adequate result. A flap can be

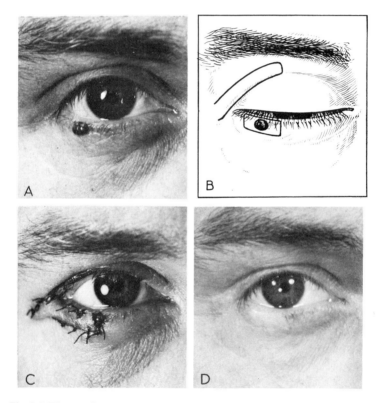

Fig. 9.6 The use of a single pedicled flap from upper eyelid in covering the defect left after excising a pigmented papilloma near the lid margin.

A   The lesion.
B   The flap outlined.
C   The flap transferred.
D   The final result after excision of the bridge segment.

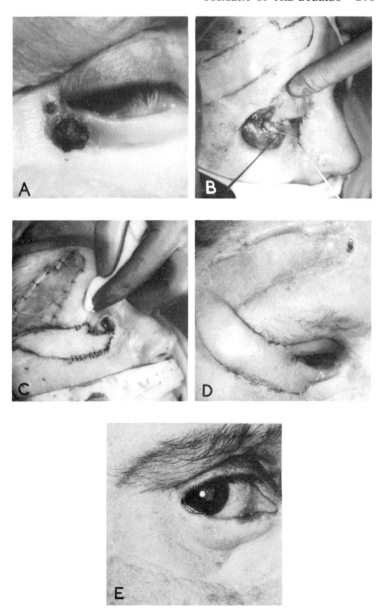

Fig. 9.7 The use of a temporal bridge pedicle to provide cover after excision of the recurrence of a basal cell carcinoma in the centre of a previously applied post-auricular whole skin graft.

    D   The lesion

    B   The excision leaving conjunctival lining, and the temporal flap outlined.

c and d   The flap transferred with secondary defect split-skin grafted.

    E   The final result after return of bridge segment of flap.

most useful, however, in the awkwardly placed simple lesion whose excision leaves a defect. Papillomata near the lid margin, for example, often require more than minimal clearance to prevent recurrence and leave a raw area which cannot readily be closed by direct suture.

Lower lid defects are particularly amenable to flap repairs and the results are functionally excellent because the bulk of eyelid movement is by the upper eyelid and a localised deficiency of orbicularis has little effect on function. When the defect does not extend beyond the eyelid on to the cheek a flap of skin from the upper eyelid above the upper palpebral furrow can be used (Fig. 9.6). The vascularity of the region permits a flap of quite outrageous length-breadth ratio to be used and depending on the length, site, etc., of the defect the flap may be used with a single pedicle at either canthus or swung down as a bipedicled strap flap. When the defect does not extend to the canthus, the flap may be used as a bridge pedicle and the unused segment, which very rapidly tubes itself, can either be returned to its donor site or excised, whichever is more convenient. These repairs are most often needed in the older age groups and the added laxity of the upper eyelid which so often goes with age makes closure of the secondary defect easier. If the secondary defect can be closed by direct suture without producing ectropion, this is the course to pursue. If not, a split-skin graft must be used.

A minor annoyance with this flap is its tendency in its early postoperative phase to become convex along its length (Fig. 9.6c) instead of remaining quite flat. Although flattening eventually takes place the convexity does detract initially from the appearance and it can be prevented by using a light-tie-over dressing of flavine wool for the flap. This produces a mild degree of concavity which flattens out on removal of the dressing.

When the defect extends beyond the confines of the lower lid a broader flap is needed and the forehead is the usual source; for the medial canthal region a glabellar type of flap can be used (Fig. 6.17); for the lateral canthus and the remainder of the lower lid a temporal flap is suitable (Fig. 9.7).

There is a moderate amount of skin available in the upper eyelid for closure by direct suture without producing ectropion and flaps are less often needed.

10

Maxillofacial injuries

The maxillofacial bony complexes are the **mandible, maxilla, malar,** and **nose,** the last three constituting the **middle third of face** (Fig. 10.1). These complexes roughly correspond to their anatomical counterparts and each has its own distinctive injury patterns. While a pattern may occur alone several patterns of fracture may exist together either in a single bony complex or in more than one at the

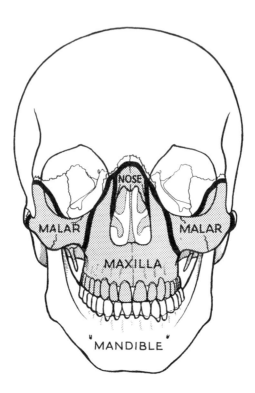

Fig. 10.1 The maxillofacial bony complexes—maxilla, nose, malars, mandible. The stippled segment indicates the middle third of face.

same time. For example a fractured maxilla may occur alone or along with fractures of one or both malars and/or nose. In either case it is loosely described as a **middle third fracture**.

In fractures of mandible and maxilla it is not uncommon for teeth to be loosened, quite apart from those in the line of the main fracture and these are described as being **alveolar fractures** because they are due to localised fractures of the alveolar plates of maxilla or mandible in relation to the loosened teeth.

Fractures of the facial skeleton can be grouped into those, like malar and nose, which do not involve the dental occlusion and those, like mandible and maxilla, where the normal occlusion of the teeth is disturbed by the fracture (Fig. 10.2).

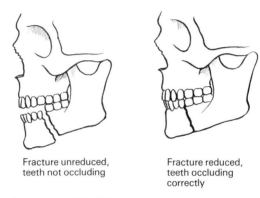

Fracture unreduced,
teeth not occluding

Fracture reduced,
teeth occluding
correctly

Fig. 10.2 In a fractured mandible if the teeth are not occluding correctly the fracture is displaced. Correct occlusion means that the fracture is reduced.

It should be appreciated at the outset that the provision and maintenance of proper dental occlusion is the core of all treatment of fractures which involve the teeth and the surgeon who has to cope with such a fracture in the absence of dental help will go far to prevent permanent and largely irreparable deformity if he makes wiring of the teeth of the upper and lower jaws together in correct occlusion the first step of local treatment.

EARLY CARE

Before their definitive treatment is begun the great majority of patients with maxillofacial injuries require no special care of the fracture other than adequate and repeated cleansing of the mouth. Mandibular fractures apart, maxillofacial fractures do not tend to be sufficiently mobile to make pain from this source a problem in early management. Even with mandibular fractures discomfort due to mobility of the fracture is seldom marked and a surprisingly small proportion require the support of a barrel bandage (Fig. 10.3).

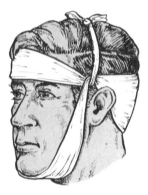

Fig. 10.3 Barrel bandage, used when necessary to support mandibular fractures.

In the small group who require special care the difficulties are either **respiratory** or caused by **haemorrhage**.

Haemorrhage
Bleeding, particularly in maxillary fractures, may occasionally be brisk but usually stops spontaneously if a free airway is provided. It is important to prevent blood from trickling back into the pharynx where it is liable to create respiratory difficulties with consequent restlessness which in turn increases the bleeding. The positioning of the patient to prevent this is described below.

Respiratory difficulty
This can vary greatly in severity and is due either to swelling of the tongue from haematoma spreading from a mandibular fracture or to inability to control the tongue in those bilateral mandibular fractures where the anterior fragment which carries most of the muscular attachments of the tongue is mobile.

The measures required in any particular patient depend on the severity of the respiratory embarrassment but *adequate suction should always be available*. Such patients breathe more easily if they can be sat up but when this is not possible it is most important not to leave them lying flat on their backs. The correct position is prone with head turned to the side (Fig. 10.4). A suture through the tongue to hold it forward may be necessary.

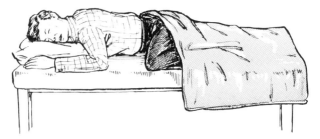

Fig. 10.4 Nursing the maxillofacial injury prone with the head to one side.

It must be stressed, however, that any tendency to serious respiratory difficulty is an indication for immediate tracheotomy and this should be done early for respiratory embarrassment tends to increase rapidly. Severe and uncontrollable bleeding may call for ligation of the external carotid artery.

ASSOCIATED INJURIES

Maxillofacial fractures do occur as isolated injuries but with car and motorcycle accidents as a common cause other injuries are very liable to be sustained sumultaneously. The injuries most likely to affect the management of the maxillofacial component are **soft tissue facial injuries, cranial injuries, chest injuries**, and **eye injuries**.

Injuries other than these interfere less significantly with the treatment of the maxillofacial fracture and the only difficulty which is apt to arise, other than that of co-operating with the orthopaedic surgeon to reduce the number of anaesthetics by working on face and limb in a single operating session, is the administrative one of deciding whether to treat the patient in orthopaedic or maxillofacial unit. Ideally he should be treated in an accident centre with the appropriate specialties converging on him but this ideal is not found universally and the situation has usually to be resolved by considering the relative severity of the several injuries.

Soft tissue facial injuries

The soft tissue injury should be treated on its own merits with the minimum of delay along the lines discussed in chapter 1. Its management is seldom significantly influenced by the simultaneous presence of a maxillofacial fracture. Even when the fracture is compound the wound can be closed with safety. Fixation of the fracture, as will be explained later, is usually via the teeth or by the alveolus itself if the patient is edentulous and so the soft tissue closure very rarely interferes with the definitive fracture treatment.

Exceptionally, when an interosseous wire (see p. 296) is used to fix the fracture in addition to the dental fixation it may be possible to use the soft tissue laceration for the surgical approach but such an occurrence is relatively rare.

Cranial injuries

Brain damage with or without a skull fracture is quite common in association with a maxillofacial injury. The unconsciousness which results affects the management of the patient in one of two ways:

1. If the patient is deeply unconscious and on this score alone would be considered for tracheotomy the presence of a fracture of maxilla or mandible with the added breathing difficulties which it causes adds great weight to the argument in favour of tracheotomy. Even where the level of unconsciousness would not by itself merit tracheotomy there should be no hesitation in carrying out one if the fracture is adding significantly to the difficulties of management and there are virtues in carrying out the procedure prophylactically rather than waiting until it becomes a therapeutic necessity. Though a tracheotomy is apt to have an unnecessary morbidity in many cases because of unsatisfactory care and poor facilities for humidifying the inspired air it can nevertheless be life saving in this situation.

2. If a tracheotomy is not considered necessary then the fitting of metal cap splints (see p. 291) and even the taking of dental impressions should be postponed until the patient is sufficiently conscious to be co-operative.

A further sign of cranial injury which may complicate the management of a maxillofacial fracture is **cerebrospinal rhinorrhoea**.

Cerebrospinal rhinorrhoea

Leakage of cerebrospinal fluid from the nose is evidence of a fracture of the cribriform plate with a dural tear. It is an easy clinical diagnosis—a water-clear fluid dropping from the nose, sometimes increased in volume by dropping the head forward or straining, usually developing within 48 hours of the injury though it may suddenly appear some days or even weeks after the injury.

The natural history of the condition if left untreated is in some dispute. Some leaks stop spontaneously when the fracture is fixed and there is no further trouble; some appear to stop but meningitis develops after a variable and sometimes quite long period of freedom from all symptoms; some continue to leak fluid with the eventual development of meningitis even after reduction and fixation of the fracture of maxilla.

It is the proportion of patients falling into each category which is disputed and this makes treatment difficult to discuss. In any case it is probably wise to enlist the help of the neurosurgeon as soon as the condition is diagnosed and all such patients should be given adequate antibiotic cover. It is well recognised that movement of the fractured maxilla causes considerable movement of the cribriform plate and the fractured neighbouring bony fragments. The fracture should therefore be reduced and fixed at the earliest possible moment so that the dural tear may get the best chance to heal.

If the leak is small in volume and becomes less fairly rapidly it can safely be left to stop spontaneously. The chances of late meningitis are probably remote.

The leak which is large in volume or which persists should be surgically closed. At a joint procedure with the neurosurgeon the dural tear is repaired with a fascial graft and the maxilla is reduced and fixed.

Chest injuries

The presence of fractured ribs along with a maxillofacial fracture does not usually complicate their mutual management. The maxillofacial injury is only likely to make treatment of the chest injury more difficult by adding to the respiratory embarrassment if there is a flail segment with paradoxical respiration. In such a situation a tracheotomy will help to solve both problems.

Eye injuries

The surprising thing about eye injuries in this context is their rarity. When one does occur the damage tends to be irreparable either with disruption of the contents of the eyeball or severe damage to the optic nerve. When damage is suspected the opinion of an ophthalmic surgeon should be sought without delay, not so much from a therapeutic point of view for there is seldom much to be done to save sight if this has already been lost but because of the possibility of sympathetic ophthalmia if the uveal tract has been damaged. The proptosis which results from bruising or actual haemorrhage into the orbital fat subsides spontaneously as does subconjunctival haemorrhage when it occurs.

Eyeball and optic nerve apart, the most frequent injury is a fracture of the orbital floor through which orbital fat may herniate into the antrum. The injury occurs usually as part of a fracture of the malar complex and will be discussed along with that injury.

REDUCTION AND FIXATION METHODS

The teeth are used as an indirect method of fixing jaw fractures. Their firm attachment to the alveolus coupled with the fact that it is their occlusion which is of prime importance from the point of view of subsequent function makes them extremely effective for this purpose. It is usually only when teeth are absent that the alveolus is approached more directly for splinting purposes.

In *reducing* a fracture of mandible or maxilla the aim is to bring the teeth of the fractured fragments into a normal relationship with those of its unfractured counterpart because the fracture must of necessity be in good position if the teeth are occluding normally. With an edentulous patient the fractured alveolus, for similar reasons, is brought into the position it would occupy if dentures were being worn.

In *fixing* a fracture of mandible or maxilla, the fractured bone once reduced must be anchored to an immovable structure. The mandible when fractured is thus anchored to the maxilla; the maxilla when fractured is anchored to the skull as well as to the mandible.

It should be appreciated in discussing the actual methods of fixation as they apply to the mandible that reduction of the fracture on to the maxilla in correct occlusion as the guide to proper reduction, and fixation to the maxilla in this position as a suitable point of anchorage are in practice achieved simultaneously because reduction and fixation are to the same structure, namely the maxilla. The separation into two distinct steps becomes more apparent with maxillary fractures where reduction is on to the mandible and fixation is to skull and mandible.

When teeth are present in sufficient numbers on both fragments they are fixed in proper occlusion by **eyelet wiring**, **arch wiring**, or **cap splinting**.

Eyelet wiring (Fig. 10.5)
The fixing device in this method is a 0.4 mm diameter length of stainless steel wire which has been doubled on itself and twisted tightly two or three times leaving a small eyelet at the end.

The double wire is passed inwards between the necks of two adjacent teeth until the twisted segment is lying between the necks with the eyelet on the outer side. The wire is then separated into its two strands, one being turned forward and one back, and each is

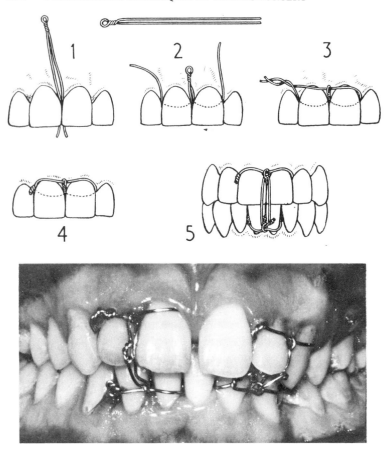

Fig. 10.5 The steps in eyelet wiring and a patient with a condylar fracture showing the upper and lower teeth wired together.

passed outwards through the next interspace so that a loop is formed round the necks of the two adjoining teeth. The loops are completed by bending the wires towards one another, passing one through the eyelet and finally twisting them tightly together before cutting off the excess and turning in the end so that it will not catch on tongue or cheek.

Several sets of these wires are applied at intervals round the alveolar arch and also at corresponding points on the opposite jaw. When the fracture has been manually reduced and the mandible closed on to the maxilla it is held in this position by looping further wires through the eyelets which oppose one another and twisting them tightly together.

Arch wiring (Fig. 10.6)

This technique is an alternative to eyelet wiring and uses a narrow malleable metal bar made of flattened soft German silver wire and accurately moulded round the alveolar arch on its outer aspect at the level of the necks of the teeth to which it is then wired. With an arch bar similarly applied to the maxilla the two can be fixed together with wires. Alternatively the arch bar on the fractured bone can be fixed to eyelet wires on the unfractured alveolus.

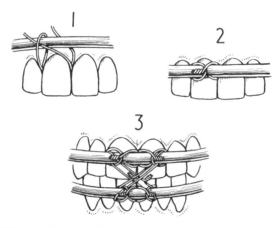

Fig. 10.6 The steps in arch wiring.

A logical development of the simple arch bar is to have hooks at intervals along its length (Fig. 10.7) so that the upper and lower bars can be more easily wired together. Various eponymous splints have been produced along those lines but they are usually referred to as **Winter-type arch bars**, the Winter's bar itself probably being the one in most common use. They are used in the same general way as the simple arch bar.

Cap splinting (Fig. 10.8)

This is much the most commonly used method in Great Britain. It is a highly developed technique in which correctly articulated models of the teeth and gums of mandible and maxilla are made in plaster of Paris. Working with these models as a basis, cast-metal cap splints are made of the entire dentition, fitting accurately over all the teeth except those purposely excluded, namely ones in the actual fracture line and those which are hopelessly carious.

Properly made and fitted these splints do no damage to gum or

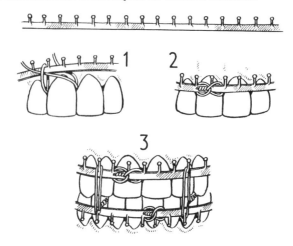

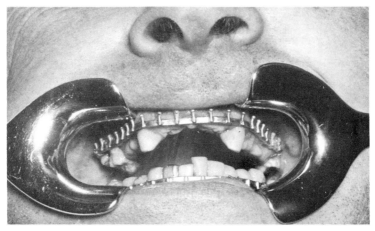

Fig. 10.7 The Winter arch bar and the steps in its application with a patient showing bars in position ready to be wired to the upper and lower teeth.

tooth and when cemented in position they provide a very positive fixation.

By planning on the articulated model it is possible to incorporate hooks at corresponding points on upper and lower splints so that the two sets of splints can be wired together or fixed with elastic bands. In this way the fractured bone can be reduced and fixed against the unfractured bone in correct position. The elastic bands are extremely useful in exerting prolonged traction when immediate reduction is not possible.

Although this describes the technique in essence there are many

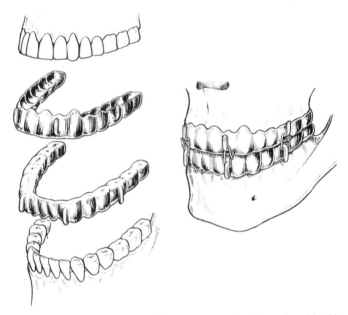

Fig. 10.8 Metal cap splints. The splints are cemented to the teeth and in this way provide fixation for a fracture of mandible or maxilla.

modifications of detail. One of these is the use of the *locking-bar* (Fig. 10.9). In this the metal cap splint is made in two sections, one on each side of the fracture line, and the mechanic in making the splints incorporates a small fitting near the adjoining end of each to permit the screwing of a connecting bar to each splint so that the sections are converted into a single rigid unit. It is not possible to have the locking bar prefabricated like the splint and instead a plaster of Paris impression is made of the fittings in their correct relative positions with the fracture reduced. A suitable bar is then made on the spot by the dental mechanic. With the bar screwed tightly in place the now single splint is wired to its fellow in the usual way. An alternative pattern of locking bar is the *Fickling dome*. It is less precise but this is regarded by some as an advantage since the fact that minor adjustments to the position of the fracture can be made when the screws are being tightened means that the entire splint, locking bar included, can be prefabricated on the plaster of Paris model.

While cap splinting is an extremely versatile technique and can be applied to all fractures of the teeth bearing segments, a problem can arise when the mandible posterior to the fracture has no teeth to provide a point of fixation—the so-called edentulous posterior

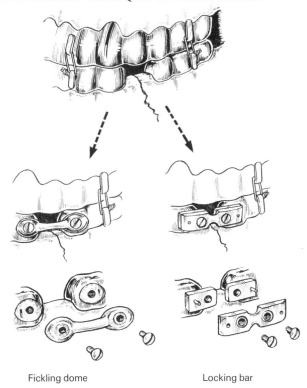

Fickling dome   Locking bar

Fig. 10.9 The two varieties of locking-bar.

fragment. In such a situation it is sometimes possible to maintain adequate reduction when displacement is minimal by extending the metal cap splint backwards through the use of a horizontal saddle (Fig. 10.10). The posterior fragment tending as it does to displace upwards and medially is in this way sufficiently well controlled.

When teeth are not present it will be appreciated that if the patient's dentures could be fitted and the fracture reduced on to the dentures with upper and lower occluding correctly the fracture would be accurately reduced. It is possible, when well fitting dentures exist, to do this but often the denture has been broken, is lost, or fits so badly as to be useless. Nevertheless the principle is still used. Impressions are taken and 'dentures without teeth', so-called Gunning splints, are made (Fig. 10.11). These splints are circumferentially wired on to the upper and lower jaws and subsequently to each other to obtain fixation (Fig. 10.12).

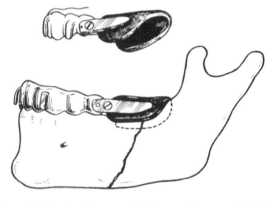

Fig. 10.10 Control of the edentulous posterior fragment in a mandibular fracture by the use of a gutta percha saddle extension of the metal cap splint.

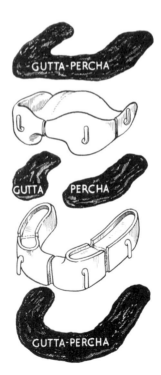

Fig. 10.11 Gunning splints, showing the gutta percha lining between the two splints and between each splint and the alveolus.

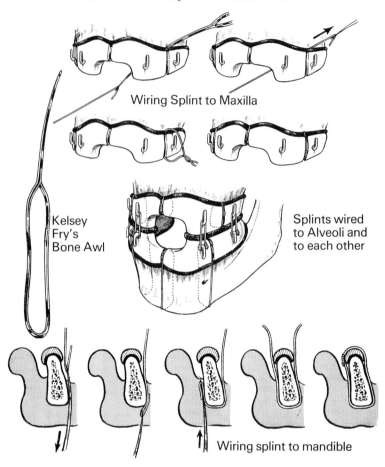

Wiring Splint to Maxilla

Kelsey Fry's Bone Awl

Splints wired to Alveoli and to each other

Wiring splint to mandible

Fig. 10.12 Gunning splints, circumferentially wired to mandible and maxilla, and to each other.

In fractures of the edentulous mandible with minimal displacement and particularly in the elderly patient it is often enough when Gunning splints have been fitted merely to support the mandible against the maxilla with a firm barrel bandage without circumferential wires. The absence of teeth makes it a little less essential to get absolutely accurate reduction for a denture can subsequently be fitted to compensate for any slight irregularity of alveolar alignment.

Internal fixation (Fig. 10.13)
When displacement of a fracture is considerable and it cannot be readily reduced manually in preparation for fixation by one of the

methods described it may be necessary to fix the bones in a reduced position by interosseous wiring or rarely by inserting a small plate.

Exposure of the mandible, necessary if internal fixation is being used, can be by an internal approach, or an external approach using a submandibular incision. This carries with it the danger of injury to the branch of the facial nerve to the lower lip, quite apart from the inevitable scar, minimal though it may be. The intra-oral approach has none of these drawbacks though the technique of wiring has to be modified somewhat. It is being increasingly used.

With the internal approach, upper border wiring is most often used. The fracture site is exposed, holes are drilled near the upper border of the mandible immediately adjoining the fracture site and a simple loop is inserted. With the fracture reduced, the wire is twisted tight to maintain reduction (Fig. 10.13). Alternative patterns of wiring can be used to maintain more effective fixation depending on the direction of the fracture.

Lower border wiring, which has been to some extent superseded by these other methods, usually makes use of a figure of eight wire and really requires an external approach. It is ideal when there is an appropriate soft tissue laceration. In such circumstances plating (Fig. 10.13) may also be possible if there is no comminution and the fracture is not too oblique, though many feel that to bury such a quantity of metal is to invite infection.

A plate may be used successfully as the sole means of bony fixation but it must be stressed that a wire by itself is not relied on to fix a fracture. Its purpose rather is maintain reduction while the metal cap or Gunning splints provide fixation in the usual way.

Infection around a wire which is well covered by the soft tissues is not common and it is usually left permanently buried. Of course infection of a mandibular fracture does occur occasionally but when one considers how many such fractures are compound into the mouth from the outset, through a tooth socket in the line of fracture, the remarkable thing about infection is its rarity. The use of a well-buried interosseous wire probably does not significantly increase the likelihood of infection. If infection does occur, the wire or plate must be removed but it should, if possible, be retained until the fracture is 'sticky' so that displacement will not recur. The upper border wire is exceptional; it is so close to the underlying mucosa that it usually becomes exposed in the mouth eventually, but removal under local anaesthesia is straightforward.

Skull fixation

The point has already been made that while the fractured maxilla is

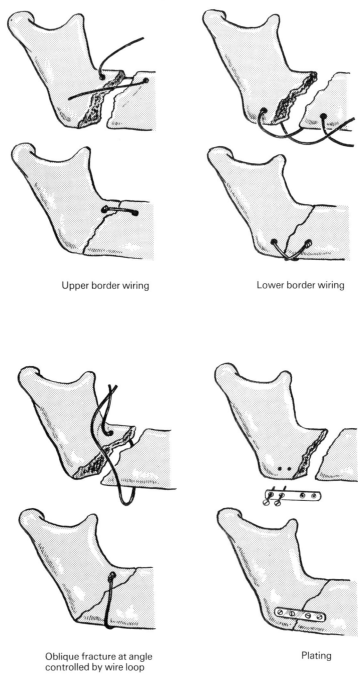

Upper border wiring

Lower border wiring

Oblique fracture at angle
controlled by wire loop

Plating

Fig. 10.13 The various methods of internal fixation of mandibular fractures.

reduced on to the mandible in good occlusion, the final anchoring fixation is to the skull. This is provided by halo fixation or supra-orbital pins.

The halo (Fig. 10.14A) consists of a circular metal band fixed by self-tapping screws into the hard outer table of the vault of the skull where it provides anchorage.

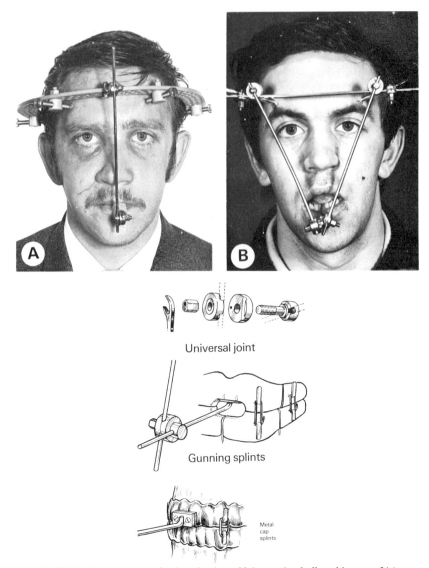

Universal joint

Gunning splints

Metal
cap
splints

Fig. 10.14 Using a system of rods and universal joints to the skull, making use of (A) a halo, (B) supra-orbital pins.

Supra-orbital pins (Fig. 10.14B). In this method a rod with a self-tapping screw at one end is inserted into the hard cortical bone of each supra-orbital ridge to provide fixed points for anchorage.

To the solid base provided by one or other of these methods, the maxillary splint, metal cap or Gunning, is fixed by a series of rods connected by universal joints. When the fracture has been reduced and the splints wired together the final fixation is achieved by tightening the universal joints to make the whole system of rods quite rigid (Fig. 10.14).

Cap splints as a method of fixation can of course only be considered when facilities are available for their construction and the alternative methods, arch and eyelet wiring, are the mainstays of treatment in many countries for treating mandibular fractures. Similarly for middle third fractures modified methods have to be employed using such techniques as the open reduction and direct interosseous wiring of fragments and fixation of the maxilla by wires to a part of the facial skeleton not involved in the fracture, e.g. the zygomatic process of the frontal bone (see p. 325).

Indeed, open reduction and wiring is being increasingly used as a method of fixation and it does have the great advantage of providing a direct visual method of fracture control. These *direct wiring methods* are discussed on page 325 *et seq*.

MALAR

Patterns of injury

There are three main types of fracture (Fig. 10.15).

Simple fracture. The fractured bone, consisting of the malar complex, remains in a single piece which is displaced medially and backwards, often tilted either medically or laterally, and usually impacted. The line of fracture runs from the infra-orbital foramen downwards and laterally over the anterior wall of the antrum compressing the infra-orbital nerve and tearing the branches of the superior dental nerve which cross the fracture line.

Comminuted fracture. The fracture pattern is generally similar to that of the simple fracture but the bone is comminuted with depression of the orbital floor. A comminuted fracture of the floor of the orbit with depression of the floor and escape of some of the orbital contents into the antrum may occur as an isolated injury—the *blow-out fracture*. Classically it results from direct force by a blunt object, e.g. a fist, on the eyeball. The loss of the orbital fat is responsible for the main clinical feature, namely enophthalmos.

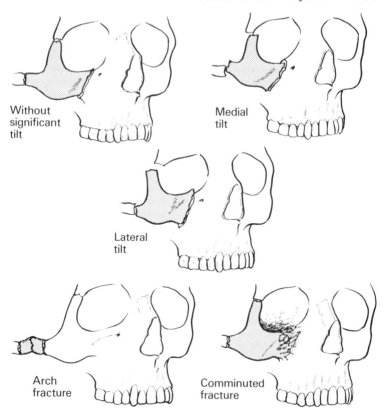

Without
significant
tilt

Medial
tilt

Lateral
tilt

Arch
fracture

Comminuted
fracture

Fig. 10.15 The types of malar fracture.

Arch fracture. This consists of a localised depression of the zygomatic arch. In its medially displaced position it tends to impinge on the coronoid process of the mandible.

Clinical picture

The clinical picture can be related very closely to the pathological anatomy of the fracture (Fig. 10.16).

Swelling and bruising of the overlying soft tissues is very variable. Sometimes it is almost completely absent, sometimes it progresses rapidly until it is severe enough to virtually close the eye and mask any underlying bony deformity. Subconjunctival haemorrhage is not uncommon.

Alteration of bony contour is usually in the direction of flattening of the cheek prominence. Comparing the inferior orbital margin with the normal on the opposite side a step in the vicinity of the infra-orbital foramen can readily be felt as a rule. If the overlying

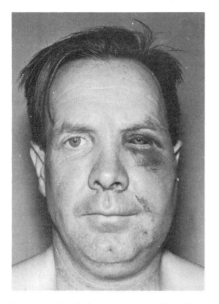

CLINICAL FEATURES
1. Soft tissue swelling and bruising
2. Flattening of cheek prominence
3. Anaesthesia of upper lip and upper teeth
4. Diplopia
5. Trismus

Fig. 10.16 Typical appearance produced by fracture of malar, and the associated clinical features.

soft tissue swelling is severe enough however it may be very difficult to detect the step. It is sometimes possible to feel the line of the fracture in the upper buccal sulcus as it runs downwards and laterally over the anterior wall of the antrum.

Anaesthesia of the structures supplied by the nerves injured is readily detected. Branches of the superior dental nerves may be divided by the fracture making the teeth of the affected segment anaesthetic to percussion. The extent of the area made anaesthetic by the damage to the infra-orbital nerve is very variable but the two areas most noticeably affected are the upper lip and the alar region of the nose. The sensory loss can vary from mild paraesthesia to complete anaesthesia and in practice it is best to ask the patient to compare the affected area with a corresponding point on the normal side.

The actual mechanism of injury to the nerve is not explicable on the basis of neuronotmesis, axonotmesis, etc., for in some patients recovery begins on regaining consciousness after the anaesthetic. In such cases recovery is invariably speedy and complete. In others recovery is slow and incomplete and one presumes that in those the injury has severely damaged or even completely divided the nerve in the infra-orbital canal.

Diplopia may occur as a transient phenomenon in the simple fracture and temporal reduction cures it. When it persists postoperatively it is usually found that the lateral part of the orbital floor has been severely comminuted and depressed. The upper visual field tends to be predominantly affected. The precise cause is not completely understood but it is thought to be due to damage to the sling mechanism of the eyeball from fibrosis and adhesions to the damaged orbital floor.

Trismus is very variable and tends to be more severe if there is much depression of the zygomatic arch. Indeed, apart from the clinically obvious local depression, trismus with marked restriction of lateral movement of the mandible may be the patient's sole complaint in the localised arch fracture.

The clinical picture of the malar fracture can be very variable indeed according to the severity of the fracture and probably the most useful single diagnostic point is the presence of infra-orbital anaesthesia. Every patient with a 'black eye' should be tested for diminution of infra-orbital sensation and a positive finding is presumptive evidence of a fractured malar.

X-ray diagnosis

The view used routinely is the 30° *occipitomental projection*—the 'sinus view', but minor degrees of displacement can be demonstrated more readily by increasing the tube angle and consequently the obliquity of the view up to 60°. The points to look for are irregularities or definite fracture lines near the infra-orbital foramen, the zygomatic arch, and the lateral wall of the antrum, and the line of the orbital floor should be compared with the normal side. Blood in the antrum may make it appear opaque.

Treatment

The finding of a malar fracture on an X-ray plate does not always mean that surgical treatment of the fracture is necessary. The need or not for surgery is decided rather on the clinical examination.

The presence of infra-orbital nerve anaesthesia, trismus, diplopia, obvious flattening of the cheek prominence—all of these are an indication for surgery. Anaesthesia of the teeth by itself is not an indication as the elevation of the malar will make no difference to this symptom. It is the case where the slightest suggestion of flattening of cheek is the only clinical finding that can cause difficulty and whether or not the fracture needs to be reduced must be an individual decision, one which incidentally can reasonably be shared with the patient. But it must be stressed that the decision to treat or not must be made as early as possible. There is no place for a 'wait and see' approach. These fractures fix in their impacted position with great rapidity and the chances of reducing a fractured malar more than a few days old are not good and become much poorer as the days pass.

Another difficult group is the one with an undisplaced fracture or even an apparently normal X-ray, but with infra-orbital anaesthesia. It is my practice to 'elevate' these malars even although no actual movement of the malar is felt because once treated recovery of sensation is uniformly rapid and complete. Many of these would doubtless recover sensation spontaneously but there is the remote possibility of the non-recovering nerve developing a very distressing and intractable neuralgia. Though the incidence of this complication is probably very small indeed the simplicity of surgical treatment makes it preferable to taking the risk of a possible late neuralgia if the fracture is left untreated.

Surgical treatment consists of elevation and this is achieved either by a **temporal approach** or by opening the antrum intraorally and inserting an *antral pack*. The temporal approach is suitable for most of the simple fractures. The deciding factor is really whether or not the malar is more or less in a single piece and capable of being reduced by exerting leverage on the anterior part of the zygomatic arch. The arch fracture of course falls into this group. When the fracture is comminuted to lever the arch would naturally only reduce part of the bone and because of this it has to be reconstituted and supported by an antral pack. There is a further small group where the fracture after a temporal reduction tends to redisplace and it is sometimes necessary to pack these also.

Following reduction most fractures maintain their reduced position but if displacement tends to recur direct *interosseous wiring* of the bones may be necessary. Wiring may also be used in conjunction both with temporal elevation and antral packing.

Temporal reduction (Fig. 10.17)
This method depends on the anatomical fact that while the temporal fascia is attached along the zygomatic arch the temporalis muscle runs under it and a lever inserted between fascia and muscle can slide down deep to the arch to exert its leverage.

With the hair shaved for 2.5 cm or so back from the temple an oblique 2 to 2.5 cm incision is made as far deeply as the temporal fascia taking care in placing it to avoid the superficial temporal vessels. It is worth pausing with retractors in the wound at this point to positively identify the fascia before incising it in the same direction and for the same length as the skin. There is often a vessel

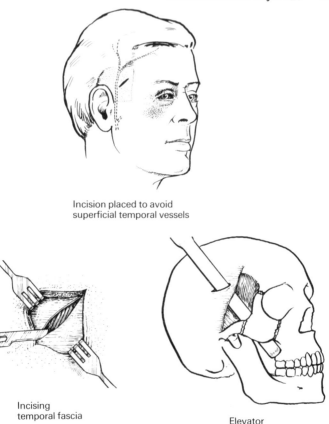

Incision placed to avoid
superficial temporal vessels

Incising
temporal fascia

Elevator
inserted

Fig. 10.17 Temporal reduction of a malar fracture.

running on the deep surface of the fascia and it is advisable to cut
carefully under direct vision. As a pathfinder for the lever
McIndoe's scissors are inserted under the fascia and slid along the
surface of the temporalis muscle deep to the zygomatic arch.

Various levers have been devised and used to elevate the bone but
the most commonly available and an eminently satisfactory one is
the orthopaedic Bristow's periosteal elevator. It is slid along the path
found by the scissors and once under the arch it should be brought
as far forward as the arch allows so that leverage can be exerted
anteriorly if necessary as well as laterally. If added leverage is
required a swab may be placed between elevator and scalp. The
degree of force needed depends on the degree of impaction and the
delay in treatment but considerable force can safely be used. In
closing the incision it is only necessary to suture the skin.

Antral reduction (Fig. 10.18)

An incision is made in the upper buccal sulcus in the canine region and the soft tissues are stripped off the outer wall of the antrum. In the type of malar fracture requiring a pack there is usually comminution of the wall and the index finger can be put straight into the antrum. When the opening is too small bone can be nibbled away to allow easy finger access. If as very rarely happens the particular part of the antral wall is intact an opening must be chisellled into the antrum and enlarged with rongeurs for access.

The finger in the antrum carefully pushes out the walls to a correct position and the most important wall is the orbital floor. The cavity is then packed with 1-inch (2.5 cm) ribbon gauze soaked in Whitehead's varnish (Pig. iodoformi Co., B.P.C.) and tightly wrung out. The striking feature of such a pack is the way it is found as clean, dry, and non-smelling on removal as when inserted. Enough packing is inserted to maintain the orbital floor at its correct level and buttress out the cheek prominence. The end of the gauze is left protruding into the mouth to give an easy start for its removal in 10 to 14 days. It is usual though not essential to partly suture the mucosal incision.

It is important not to pack too vigorously towards the orbit in case some of the pack gets pushed into the orbit itself giving rise to severe proptosis. If such an occurrence is suspected an X-ray should be taken and if it confirms the diagnosis the pack must be removed immediately and a fresh one inserted with great care. Patients with antral packs almost always develop a mild diffuse swelling of the cheek and this only subsides slowly after the pack is removed. It requires no treatment other than reassurance.

Interosseous wiring (Fig. 10.19)

The fractures are exposed with small incisions in a skin fold or wrinkle directly overlying, one in the lower eyelid and one over the zygomaticofrontal fracture line. With the bone exposed subperiosteally holes are drilled on each side of the fracture site and wiring is carried out with a simple loop or figure of eight as dictated by the local situation. The wires are left buried permanently.

When there is comminution of the orbital rim more than one wire may be needed but such wires will not of course correct any coincident depression of the orbital floor. For this antral packing may still be necessary.

It is not always essential to wire both the orbital rim and zygomatico-frontal fracture sites. Sometimes wiring of the zygomaticofrontal fracture alone combined with temporal reduction is

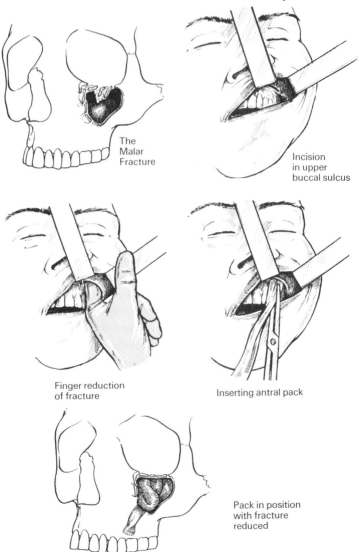

The Malar Fracture

Incision in upper buccal sulcus

Finger reduction of fracture

Inserting antral pack

Pack in position with fracture reduced

Fig. 10.18 Reduction of a fractured malar by the antral approach and maintenance of reduction by an antral pack.

adequate. The way in which interosseous wiring of the malar is used in middle third fractures is described on page 326.

Diplopia occasionally persists after elevation and the incidence of this rather distressing complication is highest when the lateral part of the orbital floor has been severely comminuted. It may also follow a blow-out fracture and on clinical examination there is limitation of

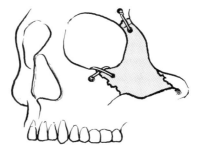

Fig. 10.19 Reduction and fixation of a fractured malar by interosseous wiring.

upward movement of the eyeball due to tethering of the inferior rectus muscle. In such circumstances exploration of the orbital floor may be needed to free the tethered rectus, return the herniated tissue to the orbit and restore the integrity of the orbital floor using a bone or cartilage graft.

If these measures fail orthoptic exercises can sometimes help in re-educating eye movements.

NOSE

Patterns of injury
The nose consists not merely of the nasal bones but also of the nasal septum and both may be damaged. Fractures follow two patterns due to **lateral** violence and **head-on** violence (Fig. 10.20).

Lateral violence. The nasal bone on the side of the injury is fractured and displaced towards the septum, the septum is deviated or fractured, and the nasal bone on the side away from the injury is fractured and displaced away from the septum so that the upper part of the nose as a whole is deviated. Depending on the severity of the violence one or more of these displacements may be present and the degree of comminution is very variable.

Head-on violence. This gives rise to saddling of the nose and broadening of its upper half as a result of the depression and splaying of the fractured nasal bones. Such a displacement naturally cannot take place without severely damaging the septum and this takes the form of gross buckling of the septum or actual septal fracture. Dislocation of the lower attachment of the septal cartilage with buckling of its columellar margin usually gives rise to deviation of the nose towards its tip.

Clinical picture
The clinical appearance of the nose and septum is the index of

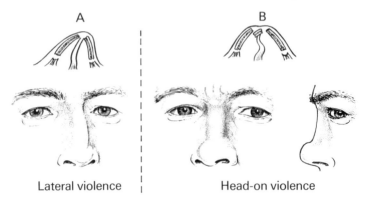

Fig. 10.20 Patterns of nasal fracture.
A   Pattern from lateral violence.
B   Pattern from head-on violence.

diagnosis. Some swelling is inevitable in patients in whom the diagnosis is being considered but a change of bridge contour or a new asymmetry are diagnostic and frequently the best judge of this is the patient himself. In any case a fractured nose, apart from its septal element, is treated on the grounds of appearance alone and an X-ray showing a fracture is of no significance unless there is associated nasal deformity.

Even when the nose is not appreciably deviated or depressed the septum should be examined for haematoma. This shows with gross bulging of the septal mucosa and it may either be unilateral or bilateral.

X-ray diagnosis
The fracture is treated on the basis of the clinical examination and X-rays are quite unnecessary.

Treatment
Nasal fractures requiring reduction should be treated with the minimum of delay for they tend to fix in their displaced position in a matter of days. The surgical approach depends on whether the fracture has resulted in **deviation** or **collapse** of the nasal bones.

Deviation
This type of displacement is caused by lateral violence and it can sometimes be corrected by simple thumb pressure (Fig. 10.21) particularly if the fracture is very recent. Unfortunately this man-oeuvre is apt to leave untouched the side depressed by the fracture

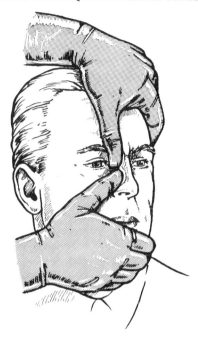

Fig. 10.21 Reduction of a nasal fracture by simple thumb pressure.

and reduces only the nasal bone which has been pushed out. Manipulation from inside using Walsham's nasal forceps is then required (Fig. 10.22). With the particular forceps for the side of the nose being manipulated the slim blade is inserted into the nostril and the broader blade outside. The blades are closed over the nasal bone which is then mobilised with a rocking movement of the forceps first laterally and then medially to disimpact it. *It is important to cover the limb of the forceps pressing on the skin with rubber tubing to protect it from undue local pressure.* With both bones mobilised finger manipulation can mould them into a symmetrical position. The septum should be inspected and if necessary reduced into a central position using Walsham's septal forceps as described below. In practice reduction of the nasal bones frequently reduces the septal displacement simultaneously.

Collapse
This displacement is the result of head-on violence and it is essential from the point of view of treatment to recognise that the nose cannot collapse without either buckling of the septum or fracture, and

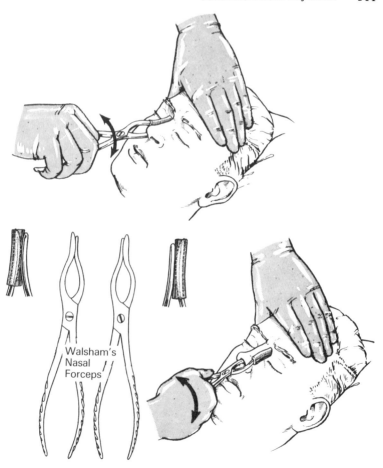

Fig. 10.22 Method of manipulating a nasal fracture using Walsham's nasal forceps. Note the use of rubber tubing to protect the skin from undue local pressure.

straightening or reconstitution automatically corrects the nasal collapse. Walsham's septal forceps are most effective for this purpose. The blades of the tightly closed forceps are so made that they remain apart leaving a gap corresponding to the thickness of the septum. With a blade inserted into each nostril along the nasal floor the forceps are 'closed' and swung up towards the nasal bridge (Fig. 10.23). As they move upwards the blades straighten the septum or reduce any fractures. The correction is completed as they reach the bridge and lift the whole bridge line forward from its collapsed position. The manoeuvre can be repeated if necessary when correction is only partial at the first attempt. Any associated broadening of

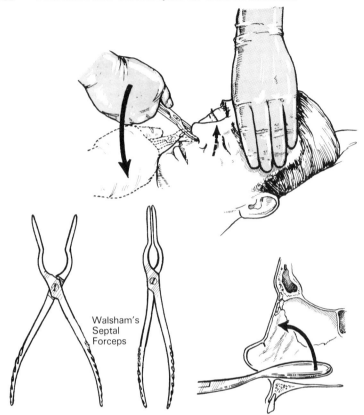

Walsham's
Septal
Forceps

Fig. 10.23 The use of Walsham's septal forceps to straighten the nasal septum.

the nasal bones can be reduced by finger pressure if necessary after mobilisation with Walsham's nasal forceps.

Septal haematoma
In a nasal injury the state of the septum is as important as that of the nasal bones and its management has been described. It should also be examined for haematoma which if present can be evacuated by incising the mucosa.

Packing and immobilisation
Tulle gras packing of the nostrils is advisable if there is the slightest mobility of the nasal bones or septum after manipulation. On the one hand it provides support for the septum in its reduced position and helps to prevent the occurrence or recurrence of haematoma. On the other it provides some counter pressure for the plaster of Paris

immobilising the nasal bones and prevents them from collapsing inwards. It can be removed in 48 hours.

A plaster of Paris splint moulded to the nose (Fig. 10.24) should be left in place for a week and worn at night for a further week or so.

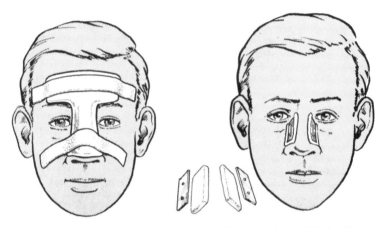

Fig. 10.24 Methods of fixing the fractured nose, by use of plaster of Paris splintage and, in the case of the grossly comminuted fracture, by the use of a through and through suture.

Particularly when it occurs as part of a severe middle third fracture the comminution of the nasal bones may be so gross that the fragments cannot be maintained in a narrow and forward position with splint and packing alone. A through and through suture tied lightly to prevent cutting-in with postoperative oedema over a strip of padded metal or rubber tubing (Fig. 10.24) is very useful in such circumstances and can be pulled forward against the rods attaching the intra-oral splint to the halo or supra-orbital pins.

When a particular fracture is seen too late for primary reduction or when the result of reduction is unsatisfactory the nose should be left until all reaction has settled when a formal endonasal rhinoplasty can be considered.

MANDIBLE

Patterns of injury

The sites of fracture (Fig. 10.25) are **condylar neck, angle, body near mental foramen, symphysis**. Fractures at these sites may occur singly or in several common combinations, namely **both condyles, both angles, body and opposite angle, body and opposite condyle, both sides of body** (Fig. 10.26).

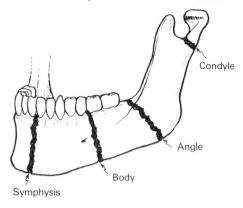

Fig. 10.25 The common sites of fracture of the mandible.

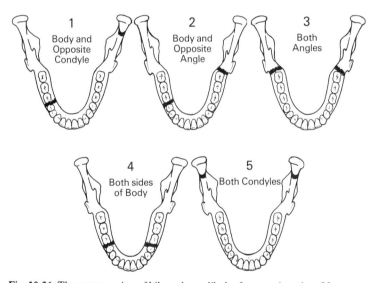

Fig. 10.26 The common sites of bilateral mandibular fractures in order of frequency.

While the displacements may be the result of the direction of the violence they depend largely on muscle pull. The muscles which elevate the mandible—masseter, medial pterygoid, temporalis—are all inserted behind the first molar; the muscles which depress the mandible—geniohyoid, mylohyoid, digastric—are all attached in front of the first molar (Fig. 10.27). Consequently the most common displacement of a posterior fragment is upwards and of an anterior fragment downwards, though the direction of the fracture line, particularly near the angle, may considerably influence the amount of displacement, either permitting or preventing it (Fig. 10.28).

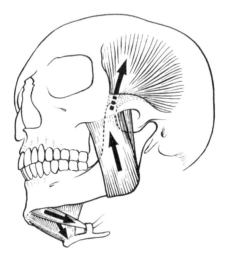

Fig. 10.27 The lines of muscle pull which influence displacement of fragments in mandibular fractures.

Upwards—masseter, temporalis, medial pterygoid.
Downwards—geniohyoid, mylohyoid, digastric.

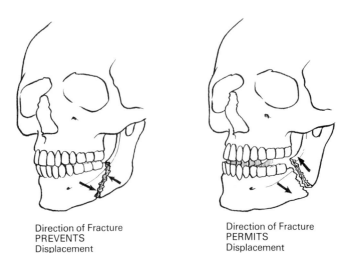

Direction of Fracture
PREVENTS
Displacement

Direction of Fracture
PERMITS
Displacement

Fig. 10.28 The effect of the direction of the fracture line on the displacement of angle fractures of mandible under the influence of muscle pull.

The condylar fracture is a special case. The condylar head is pulled forward by the lateral pterygoid muscle and when both condyles are fractured the displacement of both heads causes the patient to gag on his molars giving an 'open bite' (Fig. 10.29).

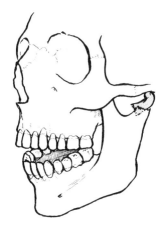

Fig. 10.29 'Open bite' produced by a bilateral condylar fracture.

Clinical picture

The site of fracture is usually indicated by swelling and local pain on movement or manipulation of the mandible. In fractures other than those of the condylar neck there is a sublingual haematoma and if the fracture is compound into the mouth there is tearing or at least bruising of the mucosa.

In the tooth-bearing segment of the mandible displacement may be clinically apparent with an obvious break in the line of the teeth or the patient may volunteer the information that 'the teeth don't close properly'.

A condylar fracture is less obvious and the only sign may be preauricular pain with or without swelling. There is restriction of movement and deviation of the mandible to the damaged side on opening with gagging of the molars on the affected side on closure. The great majority of patients with a fracture elsewhere in the mandible who complain of pain in the vicinity of the temporomandibular joint are found to have a fracture of the condylar neck.

A bilateral condylar fracture often shows clinically with an inability of the patient to close the incisors because of the gagging of the molars giving an open bite.

If the fracture is between lingula and mental foramen and there is displacement of any degree damage to the inferior dental nerve may cause anaesthesia of the lower lip. In the suspected fracture of the body a most useful method of clinical examination is bimanual intra-and extra-oral palpation, feeling along the inner and outer plates of mandible intra-orally and the lower border extra-orally (Fig. 10.30). Local swelling and tenderness is suggestive of fracture and an actual step is diagnostic.

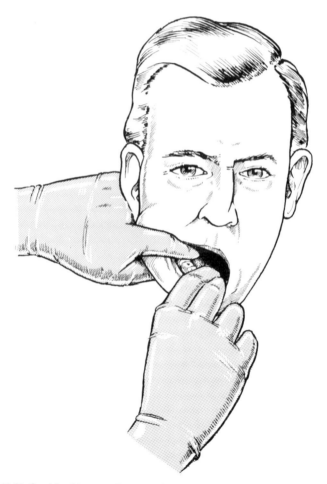

Fig. 10.30 Combined intra- and extra-oral palpation in examination of the mandible for fracture.

It is usually possible to make a fairly accurate assessment clinically but, particularly if displacement is minimal, X-ray examination may be required to confirm the diagnosis and indeed when the diagnosis is suspected X-rays should always be taken.

X-ray diagnosis

Of the possible views used to demonstrate particular parts of the mandible the two most generally useful are the **postero-anterior projection** and the **lateral oblique projection**. If further views are considered necessary the easiest way is to specify the particular parts of the bone which it is desired to demonstrate. Occlusal films are sometimes very helpful.

Treatment

When the fracture is of the tooth bearing segment treatment depends on whether the accepted routine method of dental fixation in the particular centre is by metal cap splints or whether definitive treatment is to be throughout by eyelet or arch wiring.

Where cap splinting is in common use treatment is usually by upper and lower metal cap splints or Gunning splints wired together though if displacement is minimal eyelet or arch wiring may be sufficient. If displacement is severe and manual reduction impossible dental fixation may require to be augmented by interosseous wiring. Particularly is this so if the fracture is bilateral or at the symphysis. Metal cap splints used in conjunction with interosseous wiring provide a sufficiently positive fixation but with Gunning splints circumferential wiring of the splints to mandible and maxilla is nearly always necessary. The problem of the edentulous posterior fragment is solved either by using a saddle or by interosseous wiring.

Where eyelet and arch wiring alone are used the criteria are somewhat different. The fracture with displacement minimal or nil can be handled throughout as described above by simple eyelet wires or arch bars. When gross displacement is present or the fracture is unstable, internal fixation by interosseous wiring may be necessary before the eyelet or arch wiring can be completed.

With condylar fractures no attempt is made to reduce the fragment whether or not the condyle is in the joint or dislocated. The 'joint' is treated as a pseudarthrosis and re-education of the muscles is relied on to establish good function. With a fracture of body and condyle the body fracture dictates treatment. Some patients have minimal upset with a single condylar fracture and are able to chew soft foods fairly quickly with or without a period of rest depending on the degree of initial discomfort. If pain is severe, fixation with eyelet wires or metal cap splints may be necessary for two to threee weeks. In subsequent re-education of the muscles a training flange on the splint (Fig. 10.31) may be required to train the mandible to close in correct occlusion.

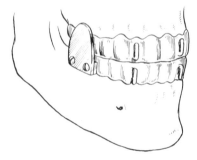

Fig. 10.31 Training flange incorporated into metal cap splint to train the mandible to close into correct occlusion.

Bilateral condylar fractures require reduction of the open bite either manually or by elastic traction on the fixing splints followed by active exercises of the mandible in two to three weeks.

Fractures other than simple condylar fractures are usually tested for union in four weeks. If there is clinical union the splints can be removed but if the fracture is still springy the splints should be wired together again until union is clinically apparent. Fractures of the symphysis and those which have become infected tend to be slow to unite. It should be recognised that X-ray evidence of union may not be present for many months.

MAXILLA AND MIDDLE THIRD

Patterns of injury

Maxilla

The fracture patterns depend on two factors—the site and direction of the violence and the anatomical lines of weakness of the maxilla. Two patterns commonly result (Fig. 10.32).

The palatal segment of the complex shears off the remainder through a horizontal line corresponding in level to the floor of the nose and the lower part of each antrum. The palate as a whole is displaced backwards and usually impacted (Fig. 10.32A).

On occasion, when the violence has been predominantly unilateral, one half of the maxilla is fractured in this way, an added fracture line running back along the midline of the hard palate. The displacement of the fractured palatal segment then tends more to be upwards with impaction into the antrum (Fig. 10.32C).

The maxillary complex is fractured as a whole. The fracture lines run upwards and medially across the anterior wall of the antrum towards the infra-orbital foramen on each side and across the nasal bones to meet in the midline at the glabellar region. Displacement is usually backwards and the inclined plane of the fracture line has the effect of forcing the maxilla also downwards, giving rise to an open bite with the patient gagging on his molars as the mandible is pushed down into an open position. The degree of impaction varies greatly from the massively displaced and impacted fracture to the so-called 'floating' fracture where impaction is minimal (Fig. 10.32B).

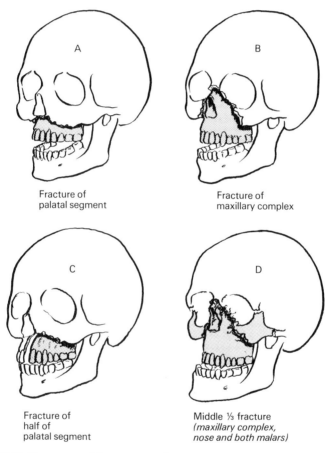

Fracture of
palatal segment

Fracture of
maxillary complex

Fracture of
half of
palatal segment

Middle ⅓ fracture
(maxillary complex,
nose and both malars)

Fig. 10.32 The common injury patterns of maxilla and middle third of face.

It must be recognised that when the maxilla is displaced in this way it is carrying the nasal complex with it. The nasal complex of course may itself be fractured independently in any of the ways already discussed.

Furthermore the maxillary fracture line passing medial to the malar corresponds to the antral line of a malar fracture and such a fracture may be present either on one or both sides along with a maxillary fracture (see *Middle third* fractures).

Middle third

While a fracture of the middle third of the face is a traumatic entity it is one which is apt to be extremely confusing because it appears to be devoid of all pattern. A pattern can readily be made to emerge as soon as it is appreciated that the fracture can be broken down into the three constituents, namely the **fracture of maxilla**, the **fracture of malars**, and the **fracture of nose** (Fig. 10.32D).

Clinical picture

Although isolated fractures of the maxilla do occur the fracture occurs sufficiently often with fractures of malar and nose that the clinical picture will be discussed under the heading of **middle third fracture**. In any case it is only after clinical examination that the actual fracture pattern can be separated from the hotch-potch of middle third fractures into the component fractures of maxilla, malar, and nose.

It is often possible to diagnose a middle third fracture on inspection alone. The face as a whole, but predominantly its middle third, is diffusely swollen with oedema of cheeks and eyelids and looks 'like a football'. It is a very typical appearance (Fig. 10.33).

In the severely displaced fracture there is an obvious 'dish-face' deformity despite the masking effect of the oedema. There is failure of the teeth to occlude properly when the patient closes his mouth. The upper incisors, instead of occluding as they do in most patients in front of the lower incisors, occlude behind or they fail to occlude at all because of the presence of an open bite. This sign is naturally difficult to elicit in the edentulous.

When there is difficulty in deciding whether any displacement of the maxillary complex is present the patient should be asked to bite on his back teeth or on his dentures if he is edentulous. If he says that the teeth are closing normally then any fracture is undisplaced.

Mobility of the maxillary complex is tested for (Fig. 10.34) by grasping the maxilla just above the incisors between finger and thumb of one hand while the other finger and thumb feel across the bridge of the nose and hold the head steady. The maxilla is rocked backwards and forwards while independent movement of maxilla is felt for. Movement of the maxilla with detectable movement at the nasal bridge suggests that the entire maxillary complex is fractured while movement of the maxilla without detectable movement at the nasal bridge suggests a fracture of the palatal segment alone. Each half of the palatal segment is then tested against the other for independent mobility and loose teeth are tested for to exclude alveolar fractures.

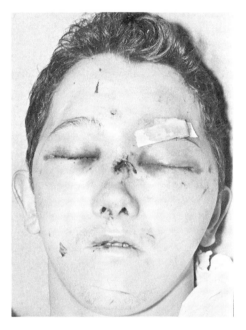

Fig. 10.33 The typical appearance of the patient with a middle third fracture.

As already stressed, middle third fractures may include fractures of either or both malars and/or nose and the presence of these must be tested for independently by the methods already indicated.

In short, maxillary fractures *per se* are diagnosed on the basis of occlusion of the teeth, and fractures of additional bones are diagnosed by actively examining the patient for their presence.

X-ray diagnosis
The diagnosis should be made on clinical examination and nearly every case can be diagnosed and treated without the need for an X-ray. In any case the interpretation of the X-ray is frequently more difficult than that of the clinical examination but the views most likely to be helpful are the 30° **occipitomental projection** and the **lateral projection**.

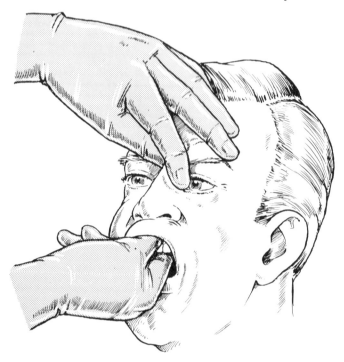

Fig. 10.34 Method of testing for mobility of the maxillary complex in a suspected middle third fracture.

Treatment

These fractures should be treated with the minimum of delay as they tend to fix rapidly in their displaced and often impacted position.

The malars to some extent and the nose completely are supported by the maxilla and it follows that they can only be properly built on a solid foundation of maxilla reduced and fixed in position. The first step then is to reduce and fix the maxilla.

If the maxilla is floating or only slightly impacted it may be possible to reduce it by finger manipulation failing which it is necessary to disimpact it with Rowe's disimpaction forceps (Fig. 10.35). Using upper and lower metal cap splints or Gunning splints wired in position the maxilla is then reduced on to the mandible and wired to the mandibular splint. It is then fixed to the particular skull fixation selected halo or pins.

The malar is then reduced, usually by the intra-oral insertion of an antral pack, sometimes with interosseous wiring. The malar fracture occurring as part of a middle third fracture tends not to be of the

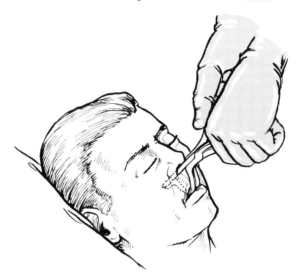

Fig. 10.35 Disimpaction of the maxilla using Rowe's disimpaction forceps. Note the downward direction of the leverage used.

variety suitable for temporal reduction, which is fortunate in view of the fact that temporal reduction can be awkward to carry out in the presence of a halo.

The fractured nose is reduced in the way already described and depending on the predominant displacement, lateral or backwards, a plaster of Paris splint or a through and through suture may be the appropriate fixation.

Where there has been a longitudinal fracture of the palate and maxillary cap splint is made in two parts with attachments for a locking-bar (see p. 293) which is applied after reduction.

The wires from maxilla to mandible providing accessory fixation can safely be removed in four weeks. Depending on the clinical assessment of union the attachment to the skull fixation is removed simultaneously or retained for a further two weeks.

Fractures of maxilla and mandible
The principle of reducing the fractured bone on to the unfractured cannot be applied straight away when maxilla and mandible are both fractured and steps must be taken to get the mandible into a reduced and rigid single unit on to which the maxilla can be reduced. This usually means the use of interosseous wiring to fix the fracture or fractures of mandible in an accurately reduced position. Reduction of the maxilla and fixation to mandible and skull can then proceed in the usual way.

DIRECT WIRING METHODS

While metal cap splints and skull fixation remain very much the standard methods of managing middle third fractures in Britain an alternative approach has been evolved in North America and other countries which does not call for elaborate dental splints and which uses a quite different mode of skull fixation. Superficially the two methods look radically different but the underlying principles are really not so very dissimilar.

In essence the method provides for the re-establishment of correct occlusion and the fixation of upper to lower alveolus by eyelet or arch wiring. This system is then fixed to an anchorage point by 'suspending' it from a point of stability on each side of the skull with a loop of stainless steel wire passing upwards through the tissues (Fig. 10.36). The most generally applicable point of stability is the zygomaticofrontal suture, though the zygomatic arch and the infra-orbital ridge have been described as possible alternatives.

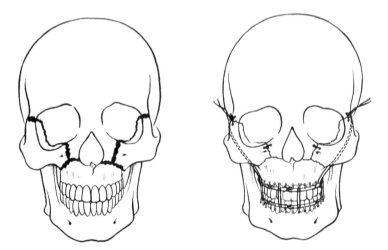

Fig. 10.36 The method of wiring the middle third fracture using interosseous wiring of fractured bones and suspension of the maxilla from the zygomaticofrontal fracture line by a wire loop (after Adams and Adams).

The details in the individual case allow of a certain amount of improvisation and this very fact is one of the advantages of the method.

Alveolar splintage.
With eyelet or Winter-type splints (p. 291) fixed to the teeth of both alveoli the fracture is reduced by the methods already described

(p. 323) and the teeth are wired together in correct occlusion. The splints can if necessary be fixed more securely by circumferentially wiring the lower splint to the mandible.

Anchorage to skull

The appropriate point to which the alveolar splints can be fixed depends on the type of fracture. In the middle third fracture (Fig. 10.32D) where fractured malars are so often part of the pattern of injury the interosseous wire reducing and fixing the zygomaticofrontal fracture line (Fig. 10.19) is used. When the fracture is of the palatal segment (Fig. 10.32A) a hole drilled through the zygomaticofrontal suture can be used or, alternatively, the suspending loop can be passed over the zygomatic arch. For this fracture the infra-orbital ridge has also been used.

Of these possible fixation points the zygomaticofrontal suture or fracture line has the obvious advantage that it can be used for almost all types of middle third fracture as well as those of the maxilla alone. As a result it is much the most frequently employed and further discussion will be restricted to describing its use alone.

Method of wiring (Fig. 10.37)

The wire loop should run as vertically as possible and this means that it should be attached to the alveolar splintage system in the vicinity of the first molar. A common error is to have the attachment too far forward so that the wire runs unduly obliquely backwards and up with a consequent tendency on tightening to increase rather than correct the open bite tilt displacement of the fractured bone (Fig. 10.32).

The loop wire can be passed through the tissues using a spinal needle, a bone awl (Fig. 10.12), or a dissecting probe.

A 0.4 mm diameter wire is passed through the zygomaticofrontal drill hole or wire loop fixing the zygomaticofrontal part of the malar fracture. The spinal needle is inserted through the mucous membrane of the upper buccal sulcus above the first molar and passed upwards behind the body of the malar towards the zygomaticofrontal suture. The two ends of the wire are threaded down the needle into the mouth and the needle is then withdrawn. Alternatively the wires are carried down to the mouth by the awl or dissecting probe. The wire is finally looped through the alveolar splint and tightened. Care should be taken not to overtighten.

With splints on upper and lower alveolus wired together it does not greatly matter whether the loop is attached to maxillary or mandibular splint. If the loop is fixed to the maxillary splint it may

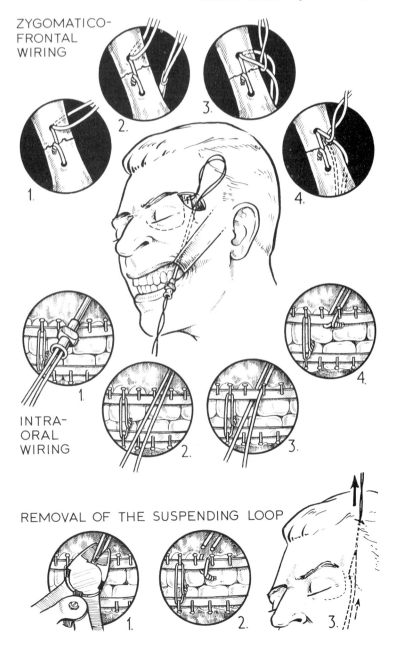

ZYGOMATICO-
FRONTAL
WIRING

INTRA-
ORAL
WIRING

REMOVAL OF THE SUSPENDING LOOP

Fig. 10.37 The stages in the application and subsequent removal of the wiring method shown in Figure 10.36. The wires fixing the Winter's splint to the teeth are omitted for clarity.

tend to pull the gum upwards off the teeth and cause trouble. This can be avoided by fixing the loop to the mandibular splint or even to the wire holding upper and lower splints in proper occlusion.

Near the anchorage point on the zygomaticofrontal suture a Bunnell-type pull-out wire is usually passed through the loop and brought out at the surface so that when the time comes to remove the wiring the loop can be cut inside the mouth and withdrawn through the temporal skin using the pull-out wire.

The method can conveniently be combined with direct exposure and interosseous wiring of comminuted fragments and will work very well as long as it is remembered that the primary object throughout is to achieve and maintain correct dental occlusion until the fracture has united.

Index

Bold type denotes illustrations on pages apart from those containing
the textual reference